Medical Genetics in the Clinical Practice of ORL

Advances in Oto-Rhino-Laryngology

Vol. 70

Medical Genetics in the Clinical Practice of ORL

Volume Editors

Raye L. Alford Houston, Tex.

V. Reid Sutton Houston, Tex.

11 figures, 2 in color and 20 tables, 2011

KARGER Basel · Freiburg · Paris · London · New York · Bangalore · Bangkok · Shanghai · Singapore · Tokyo · Sydney

Raye L. Alford
Bobby R. Alford Department of
Otolaryngology –
Head and Neck Surgery
Baylor College of Medicine
One Baylor Plaza, NA102
Houston, TX 77030 (USA)

V. Reid Sutton
Texas Children's Hospital
6701 Fannin St., Suite 1560.10
Houston, TX 77030 (USA)

Library of Congress Cataloging-in-Publication Data

Medical genetics in the clinical practice of ORL / volume editors, Raye L. Alford, V. Reid Sutton.
p. ; cm. -- (Advances in oto-rhino-laryngology, ISSN 0065-3071 ; vol. 70)
Includes bibliographical references and indexes.
ISBN 978-3-8055-9668-8 (hard cover : alk. paper) -- ISBN 978-3-8055-9669-5 (e-ISBN)
1. Otolaryngology--Genetic aspects. I. Alford, Raye L. II. Sutton, V. Reid. III. Series: Advances in oto-rhino-laryngology ; v. 70. 0065-3071
[DNLM: 1. Otorhinolaryngologic Diseases--genetics. 2. Gene Therapy--trends. W1 AD701 v.70 2011 / WV 140]
RF46.M43 2011
617.7'524--dc22

2010054257

Bibliographic Indices. This publication is listed in bibliographic services, including Current Contents®.

www.karger.com
Printed in Switzerland on acid-free and non-aging paper (ISO 9706) by Reinhardt Druck, Basel
ISSN 0065–3071
ISBN 978–3–8055–9668–8
e-ISBN 978–3–8055–9669–5

Contents

Preface

The sequencing of the human genome, completed in 2003, laid the foundation for great advances in scientific knowledge and molecular and informational technologies. Because of the Human Genome Project, which took 20 centers around the world over 5 years to complete at a cost of USD 2.7 billion, an individual's entire genome (all their genetic information) can today be sequenced for less than USD 10,000. The cost of whole genome sequencing and our understanding of the genome will continue to change exponentially, and individuals may soon have their whole genome sequenced as part of routine medical care.

There is almost no part of the clinical practice of otorhinolaryngology that is not touched by genetics. It has long been recognized that an immense number of genetic syndromes include hearing loss, craniofacial abnormalities, cochlear malformations, cleft lip/palate, and tumors of the head and neck. In recent years, the genetic causes of many of these syndromes and a number of other conditions including nonsyndromic hearing loss and chronic rhinosinusitis have been elucidated, resulting in an improved understanding of the developmental and biochemical processes involved, allowing the development of genetic tests to aid in diagnosis and risk assessment, and suggesting novel approaches for therapeutic intervention.

This book is written as a practical guide to medical genetics as it applies to the clinical practice of otorhinolaryngology. It describes recent advances in understanding the genetics of diseases of the head and neck, introduces emerging knowledge and trends, and provides resources that empower clinicians to incorporate genetics into clinical practice, thereby improving patient care.

Raye L. Alford, Houston, Tex.
V. Reid Sutton, Houston, Tex.

Alford RL, Sutton VR (eds): Medical Genetics in the Clinical Practice of ORL.
Adv Otorhinolaryngol. Basel, Karger, 2011, vol 70, pp 1–9

Genetic Basis of Conditions Commonly Seen in ORL Practice

David R. Friedmann · Anil K. Lalwani

Department of Otolaryngology, New York University School of Medicine, New York, N.Y., USA

Abstract

As science continues to unravel the genetic basis of disease, an understanding of genetics has become increasingly critical to the practicing clinician. Otorhinolaryngology, a comprehensive specialty in which the physician is responsible for delivering both medical and surgical care within their scope of practice, requires the practitioner to have a fund of knowledge in genetics to effectively communicate and counsel patients. This introductory chapter highlights what is known about the complexity of the human genome and various applications of genetics throughout the field of otorhinolaryngology to be discussed in subsequent chapters. These entities include the genetics of hearing impairment, skull base tumors, molecular genetics in head and neck cancer and systemic diseases with otolaryngologic features.

At the simplest level, the enormity and complexity of the human genome is reflected in its size: at just over 3,000,000,000 bp, it is one the largest among mammals. Stretched end-to-end, it would be 2 m in length, and yet, quite remarkably, it is folded by its secondary, tertiary, and quaternary structure to fit into the nucleus of the human cell that is only 6×10^{-8} m in diameter (table 1). Our understanding of the genome began in earnest with the elucidation of the structure of DNA in 1953 by Watson and Crick – the double helix not only identified the structure, but also explained how DNA replicated itself (table 2). The machinery for transcription (DNA to RNA) and translation (RNA to protein) was next to be deciphered. The discoveries of these mechanisms led to the observation that the fundamental working of the cell was a unidirectional flow from DNA to RNA to protein. Not long thereafter, our ignorance of the etiology of many diseases was lessened as we began to comprehend the contribution of genetics to their pathophysiology – it was at this point that the field of human genetics was born. One such example was the ability to isolate, stain and visually inspect the chromosomal content of cells by karyotyping; it was in 1959, a mere 50 years ago, when we first learned that Down syndrome was due to trisomy 21 [1].

The ability to sequence and manipulate DNA through recombinant DNA technology in the 1970s and 1980s greatly facilitated the study of specific genes and their function. Recombinant DNA technology also raised ethical concerns about our ability to manipulate the building blocks of life and its potential impact on what it means to be human; these concerns persist today as the technology and our capabilities have become even more sophisticated. The development of the polymerase chain reaction (PCR) which

Table 1. Interesting facts about the human genome

The human genome contains just over 3 billion basepairs of DNA
Humans are 99.9% identical at the genome level regardless of race
In direct sequence comparison, the chimpanzee genome differs from that of the human genome by only 1.23%
Our entire DNA sequence would fill 200 1,000-page New York City telephone directories
The total length of DNA present in one adult human is 60 trillion feet or around 10 billion miles of DNA: the equivalent distance of 59 round trips from Earth to the Sun
The human genome contains approximately 20,000–25,000 genes that code for proteins – a number much less than the 200,000 expected based on the size of the genome. This constitutes only about 1.5% of genome
The remaining genome consists of noncoding RNA genes, regulatory sequences, introns and 'junk DNA'; the latter junk DNA, whose function remains currently unknown, comprises nearly 97% of the human genome
The mitochondrial DNA has a 20-fold higher rate of mutation compared to nuclear DNA; it is only passed on by the mother from one generation to the next as it is contained in the egg, but not the sperm
The evolutionary branch between the primates and the mouse occurred 70–90 million years ago
Compared to other mammals, humans have lost a significant number of olfactory genes; consequently, our sense of smell is less complex when compared to other mammals

Table 2. A timeline of major discoveries in genetics

1860	Gregor Mendel, 'father of genetics', experiments with pea plants to define basic laws of inheritance
1910	T.H. Morgan elucidates the chromosomal basis for genetic inheritance and the principle of linkage by cross-breading fruit flies
1930	Beadle-Tatum propose 'one gene-one enzyme' theory
1940	Barbara McClintock studying maize discovers transposons or 'jumping genes'
1940s	Avery and McLeod demonstrate DNA is 'transforming factor' previously noted by Fred Griffith
1950	Chargaff's Rules of nucleic acids of one-to-one ratio of paired nucleotide bases (A-T, G-C)
1953	Watson and Crick describe double-helix configuration of DNA
1958	Meselson and Stahl prove the semiconservative method of DNA replication
1959	Karyotyping with applications to basic science experiments and the prenatal detection of disease
1960	RNA discovered, contributing to our understanding of central dogma theory
1960s	Restriction enzyme technology used to cut DNA at specific recognition sites
1970s	RNA splicing discovered
1980s	DNA fingerprinting using polymorphisms for forensic cases
1985	Polymerase chain reaction (PCR) developed to amplify small pieces of DNA
1989	Gene for cystic fibrosis on chromosome 7 identified
1990s	RNA interference used to silence targeted genes
2000s	Human genome project completed and identified ~25,000 human genes

Table 3. Complexity of the genome

Mutation in a single gene may cause both recessive and dominant disease
Digenic inheritance: disease is a result of individual mutations in two different genes
Complex inheritance: interaction of multiple genes determines the phenotype
Multifactorial inheritance: interaction of environment and several genes may determine phenotype
Genomic imprinting: a process by which the gene of one of the parents is silenced (not expressed)
Post-transcriptional modification: 5′ capping, 3′ polyadenylation, gene splicing
MicroRNA: post-transcriptional regulators that bind to complementary sequences of mRNA causing targeted gene silencing
Small-interfering RNA: double-stranded RNA molecules that function in RNA interference pathway
Post-translational modification: addition of functional groups including methylation, acetylation, formylation
Epigenetics: chemical, nonmutational modifications in DNA structure which may affect inheritance patterns
Single-nucleotide polymorphism or SNP: a single nucleotide (A, T, C or G) variation between members of a species or paired chromosome in an individual; it occurs with a frequency of 1 in 100–300 bp

allows for the generation of billions of copies of a DNA sequence of interest has been the catalyst for the next revolution in molecular genetics: gene mapping [2].

With much fanfare, the genome project was conceived and launched in the late 1980s and early 1990s to identify markers throughout the human genome that would facilitate the creation of a genetic road map of each of the chromosomes. Early successes included the identification of genes for cystic fibrosis [3] and neurofibromatosis [2, 4]; both diseases important in otolaryngology with the former associated with chronic sinusitis and the latter characterized by bilateral vestibular schwannomas. In addition, the genome project began what, at that time, seemed like a gargantuan undertaking – to sequence the human genome in its entirety (today, we can get our DNA sequenced for USD 50,000 in less than 2 weeks). Naively, many believed that once the human genome was sequenced, understanding genetics would be simple and we would finally know what aspect of our genome makes us humans and what distinguishes us from other animals. There was also the hope that we would understand the genetic factors associated with cancer, chronic diseases and aging. It was thought that with the implementation of genetic diagnosis on a large scale, we could intervene and modulate these factors to lessen the burden of human disease.

In reality, the sequencing of the human genome and that of other species has shed light on the true complexity of the genome (table 3). The complex genetic inheritance model in which many genes interact with environmental factors to cause a single disease has supplemented the single gene-single disease model. The interaction of the environment with one's genetic predisposition is being studied in diverse fields from auditory neuroscience to carcinogenesis. This work has implications for many otolaryngologic conditions such as hearing loss, head and neck cancer, and chronic sinus infections.

With the discovery of micro RNA (miRNA) and inhibitory RNA (RNAi) that regulate gene expression and translation, respectively, our concept of RNA is no longer restricted to coding for proteins. Quite remarkably, even these small nucleic acid sequences are responsible for diseases in humans – including hearing loss [5]. Clearly, the genetic machinery has layers of control and redundancy, some expected, several unanticipated, and much that is yet to be elucidated.

As otolaryngologist-head and neck surgeons, we have benefited greatly from the genetic revolution. Genetics has become increasingly important to the ear, nose and throat practitioner in the evaluation, diagnosis and treatment of many conditions and its role is certain to become even greater with further elucidation of the molecular basis for, as yet, poorly understood diseases. We look forward to a future where we will define the molecular characteristics of an individual patient's disease and design treatment that uniquely addresses their underlying problem.

The goal of this textbook is to begin this journey – to harvest the current knowledge on the genetic basis of diseases in oto-rhino-laryngology and promulgate how it might be used to better care for our patients. Basic principles of medical genetics will be reviewed with the goal of demonstrating how to begin the work up of a patient with a suspected genetic disease and how to best utilize available resources to improve the quality of care. In this chapter, we will preview select otolaryngologic conditions that are particularly illustrative of the diverse and continually expanding role of genetics in otorhinolaryngology and will be discussed further in subsequent chapters.

Genetics of Hearing Impairment

Hearing loss is the most common sensory deficit in humans and 50% of cases are believed to be related to genetics. Nonsyndromic hereditary hearing impairment (hearing loss occurring in isolation) accounts for 2/3 of cases, while syndromic hereditary hearing impairment (hearing loss in the presence of other systemic problems such as eye or kidney disease) makes up the remainder of cases. At birth, 1–4 of every 1,000 newborns have severe to profound sensorineural hearing loss. By age 75, nearly half do [6]. Despite its prevalence, there is a dearth of curative interventions; while hearing aids can amplify sound and cochlear implants can provide sufficient information for open set speech recognition, no available treatment restores, prevents, or arrests hearing loss.

Through the centuries, deciphering the molecular basis of hearing has been impeded by the unique anatomy of the inner ear: the mechanosensory apparatus is small in size, it is made up of numerous types of unique cells that cannot be grown or duplicated in the Petri dish, and it is encased in one of the hardest bones in the body, impenetrable to bullets. Thus, it is not surprising that by the mid-20th century, the protein building blocks of the inner ear remained a mystery and most hearing loss had been attributed to environmental causes. With improved antibiotic therapies and vaccinations, hearing loss as a complication of tympanomastoiditis and infections became less prevalent and hearing loss was increasingly attributed to hereditary hearing impairment. Today, it is believed that nearly half of all childhood deafness is hereditary and that age-related hearing loss or presbyacusis is genetically determined [7]. Moving forward, our conception of hearing impairment must be informed by advances in molecular genetics and understood as the interaction between genetic susceptibility and environmental influences.

Over the past two decades, there have been significant advances in our understanding of molecular genetics of deafness facilitated by the tools generated by the genome project. Genetic mapping studies of small and large families have identified over 100 loci that harbor genes for recessive, dominant and X-linked nonsyndromic deafness. These mapping studies would not have been possible without the identification of randomly distributed di- and tetra-nucleotide repeats throughout our genome flanked by unique gene sequences. Using PCR technology has allowed for the mapping of locations of nonsyndromic deafness genes. Of even greater importance, the identity of nearly half of these genes has been elucidated, aided by the availability of the human genome sequence and the catalog of genes encoded in the mapped regions. The nature and function of some of these genes were anticipated, such as cytoskeletal and structural proteins (myosins, stereocilia and tectorial proteins) and ion channels (sodium, potassium, iodine) as these were predicted to be important in sensory hair cell function. The protein products of other genes involved in nonsyndromic deafness were unexpected, including transcription factors and developmental genes which regulate morphogenesis, adhesion proteins responsible for cell to cell membrane interactions, and gap junction proteins which function in intercellular communication [8]. The latter, *GJB2* encoding Connexin 26, a gap junction protein that may play a role in potassium shuttling, may be responsible for up to half of childhood recessive deafness in some populations! A larger number of genes responsible for syndromic deafness have also been identified including those for Usher syndrome, Waardenburg syndrome and Alport syndrome to name a just a few.

There has been a paradigm shift in our understanding of the genetics of deafness. While the distinction of syndromic versus nonsyndromic deafness remains clinically important, it has now been repeatedly shown that the same gene can cause both. One example of this is the *SLC26A4* gene, encoding pendrin, in which different mutations may cause a spectrum of abnormalities from pendred syndrome to nonsyndromic hearing loss from an isolated large vestibular aqueduct, the most common inner ear malformation. Similarly, a single gene can be associated with recessive and dominant inheritance (*GJB2*, *MYO7A*). On other occasions, inheritance of deafness is associated with a mutation in two different genes, a concept called digenic inheritance (a single mutation in *GJB2* and *GJB6*) [9]. These discoveries highlight the shortcomings of previous dogma associating single genes with a particular disease phenotype.

Advances in the genetics of deafness have impacted how we evaluate children with hearing loss. In the past, the diagnostic evaluation of a child with severe to profound SNHL included a panel of laboratory tests, consultation and radiologic imaging. Now, given that *GJB2* mutations are responsible for a large percentage of childhood recessive deafness, some clinicians advocate genetic testing for mutations in *GJB2* by sequencing the entire gene as an initial step [10]; it is also recommended that mutations in *GJB6* be excluded since digenic inheritance has been demonstrated [9]. As *GJB2* deafness is most frequently nonsyndromic and is associated with a normal inner ear, other tests looking for syndromic features and radiologic abnormalities are usually not necessary. This approach of sequencing the entire gene is feasible in the case of *GJB2* because of its small size. In contrast, this is not feasible for *SLC26A4* because its large size currently makes it too expensive to screen by direct sequencing; in this case, practical considerations dictate that genetic testing be confined to screening for the known common mutations. However, as sequencing becomes fast and inexpensive, direct sequencing of all known genes for deafness or even the sequencing of a deaf individual's entire genome may replace single gene screening for hearing loss and other diseases.

Identification of the genetic etiology of hearing loss is clinically important for a child with hearing loss. For example, an infant who fails hearing screening at birth may undergo immediate screening for *GJB2* mutations; if positive, one can be certain that the child likely has severe to profound SNHL. Thus, the focus for the child who has failed infant hearing screening shifts from re-screening to establishing hearing thresholds and proceeding with intervention (hearing aids, speech therapy) at the first follow-up visit. In addition, several published studies have now demonstrated excellent rehabilitative outcome with cochlear implantation in children with *GJB2* deafness [11]; this information is critically important for parents as they make therapeutic decisions for their child. We are rapidly moving towards a future when a child with hearing loss will undergo

Table 4. Fundamental of oncogenesis

Carcinogenesis is the malignant transformation of cells leading to tumor formation
Proto-oncogenes may mutate to oncogenes: gain of function, giving these cells survival advantage (*RAS*, *EGFR*)
Tumor supressor genes normally inhibit cell growth: loss of function, often require 'two hits' for inactivation (*RB*, *BRCA-1,2*, *BCL-2*) except in cases of haplo insufficiency or dominant negative gene products (*TP53*)
Malignant cells acquire the ability for unchecked growth, loss of apoptosis, acquisition of angiogenesis capabilities and the ability to metastasize by loss of cell adhesion

genetic screening for mutations in deafness genes and will have intervention determined by both the severity of the hearing loss and its molecular etiology. Soon thereafter, molecular therapy in the form of gene therapy or stem cell therapy may become available to restore hearing, the subject of a subsequent chapter in this book.

Molecular Genetics in Head and Neck Cancer

According to the National Cancer Institute, head and neck cancers account for 3–5% of all cancers in the United States with nearly 40,000 new cases annually. Squamous cell carcinoma of the head and neck is the 10th most common cancer in the world. Common risk factors include alcohol consumption, smoking and human papillomavirus (HPV) infection. Certain rare genetic disorders may also predispose patients to develop squamous cell carcinoma of the head and neck. These include Bloom syndrome, ataxia telangiactasia, Fanconi anemia, and Li-Fraumeni syndrome. In such cases, the malignancy may arise in patients at a much younger age, be more aggressive and associated with a poorer prognosis. The 5-year survival for all stages of head and neck cancer is a dismal 35–50%, with nearly 1/3 of patients ultimately succumbing to their disease. Despite advances in treatment of head and neck cancer over the last several decades, the 5-year mortality has not diminished significantly. Much hope is currently placed on the expectation that advances in the molecular understanding of head and neck cancer will lead to novel therapies that will have a meaningful impact on patient survival.

The development of head and neck cancer is a multi-step process progressing from epithelial dysplasia to invasive neoplasia (table 4). Many different genes are involved in this transformation including those that are involved in cellular signaling, cell cycle, apoptosis, genomic stability, the cytoskeleton, and angiogenesis. Efforts have focused on defining which specific genes are turned on and which genes are turned off in carcinogenesis. Advances in molecular technology have greatly facilitated 'profiling' the gene expression of dysplastic and neoplastic cells [12]. Changes in the expression levels of over 100 genes are implicated in malignant transformation, most of which can be classified as oncogenes or tumor suppressor genes. The neoplastic cell in the head and neck is likewise characterized by overactive oncogenes or by tumor suppressor genes that have been turned off [13]. Oncogenes facilitate malignant transformation by allowing for uncontrolled cell growth whereas mutated tumor suppressor genes may lose their ability to block cell growth. For example, tumor protein *TP53* is a tumor suppressor gene whose protein product arrests the cell cycle phase thus allowing repair of genetic injury. It also induces apoptosis. HPV, a causative agent of certain types of head and neck cancer, encodes a protein that has been shown to bind TP53 leading to decreased TP53 function and subsequently tumorogenesis in vitro. Understanding the role of TP53 in oncogenesis has led to gene therapy trials that restore TP53 function thus promoting its antitumor function. Similar trials are underway with other oncogenes and tumor suppressor genes to treat cancer [14].

A greater understanding of the molecular events underlying the development of head and neck carcinoma has allowed for the stratification of patients with squamous cell carcinoma based on their gene expression profile [15]. These expression profiles and molecular markers can be used to glean prognostic information and identify those at high risk for primary and recurrent disease [16]. These biologic profiles may soon replace traditional staging tumor node metastasis (TNM) to guide treatment strategies and predict the likelihood of a therapeutic response to particular modalities. For example, the level of expression of certain tumor suppressor genes involved in regulating apoptosis (such as *BCL-2*) has been shown not only to correspond with the tumor's aggressiveness but is also predictive of the likelihood of treatment response [17].

A patient's expression profile may soon be used to design tumor and patient specific targeted therapy. It has been shown that there is upregulation of epidermal growth factor (EGF) family of receptors in cancer [18]. This finding has led to the development of monoclonal antibodies directed against EGF receptor such as Cetuximab as therapeutic agents to decrease the proliferative capacity of tumors. An active area of research is modulating the expression of genes critical in neoplasia through the use of miRNA, RNAi, or gene therapy. This research may potentially lead to prevention of malignant transformation in the first place by regulating the expression of neoplasm promoting genes.

Skull Base Tumors

Investigation of the genetics of skull base tumors such as paragangliomas and vestibular schwannomas has further highlighted the complexities of the human genome and the potential of molecular genetics to revolutionize patient care. Paragangliomas of the head and neck are rare neuroendocrine tumors of the chromaffin-negative glomus cells derived from embryonic neural crest cells, that can enlarge to cause deafness and facial palsy. Four separate genes have been identified whose mutant alleles are linked to hereditary paragangliomas all of which encode distinct subunits or modifiers of a mitochondrial protein (*SDHB, SDHC, SDHD, SDHAF2*). The inheritance pattern of familial paragangliomas due to mutations in SDHD is unusual in that it involves genomic imprinting of the maternal allele that leads to its silencing. In humans, imprinting is a common phenomenon and occurs through epigenetic modification during gametogenesies. It leads to differential expression of the parental alleles; for an imprinted gene, either the mother or father's gene is expressed in the offspring, but not both. In familial cases of paragangliomas, transmission of the disease occurs only if the mutated paraganglioma gene is passed down by the father (who does not himself have to be affected). If the mother passes down the mutated gene, the son/daughter will not develop glomus tumors. An understanding of this inheritance pattern allows for identification of at risk patients through family histories and a detailed family pedigree [19]. This information can then be used for genetic counseling and aggressive clinical and radiologic surveillance for these lesions in those at risk while avoiding unnecessary surveillance in others.

Vestibular schwannoma, also known as acoustic neuroma are the most common tumors of the cerebellopontine angle. The majority of vestibular schwannomas are sporadic in occurrence and unilateral, while only 5% are familial. The familial cases of vestibular schwannomas are most often associated with neurofibromatosis type II (NF2). The incidence of NF2 is estimated between 1 in 33,000 and 1 in 50,000 [4] and NF2 patients often present with bilateral vestibular schwannomas at a young age. NF2 is inherited in an autosomal-dominant manner and is due to mutation in the *NF2* gene coding for the protein merlin. Merlin is a tumor suppressor gene whose loss of function may contribute to tumorigenesis by disinhibition of cell growth [20]. Thus, tumor suppressor genes are important in the pathogenesis of both benign and malignant tumors. A better understanding of the molecular role of this gene in tumor formation may enable the development of novel therapies for neurofibromatosis.

Systemic Disease with Otolaryngologic Features

Certain conditions presenting to the otolaryngologist should prompt an exam for systemic findings consistent with known genetic diseases. For example, endolymphatic sac tumors are seen most often in association with Von Hippel Landau syndrome in which mutations in this tumor suppressor gene may predispose the patient to other benign and malignant tumors. Hereditary hemorrhagic telangiectasia or Osler Weber Rendu syndrome is an autosomal-dominant disorder involving genes related to transforming growth factor receptor-β (TGF-β) causing small vascular malformations that may present with otolaryngologic symptoms including spontaneous recurrent epistaxis [21]. Cystic fibrosis is the most frequent lethal autosomal-recessive disease in the Caucasian population in which approximately 1 in 25 people are carriers of a mutation. Patients with cystic fibrosis may manifest otolaryngologic symptoms including chronic sinusitis [22]. With the identification of the most common mutations, cystic fibrosis screening has become part of a battery of prenatal tests for at risk populations. Efforts have also classically been focused on using gene therapy to express the normal CFTR gene in target tissues, but with limited clinical application currently.

The pervasive role of genetics even extends to the evaluation of infectious conditions in otolaryngology such as rhinosinusitis. In cases of chronic sinusitis, genetic testing to assess for mutations may reveal an underlying etiology predisposing the patient to recurrent infections.

Conclusions

While much progress has been made in our understanding of the genetic basis of disease, there remain whole entities about which very little is understood. Otosclerosis, vestibulopathies, noise-induced hearing loss, and otitis media are a few of the otolaryngologic conditions of which we now have a rudimentary understanding of the role that genetics plays and will be discussed further in the remainder of this book.

In future chapters, this book will delve into some of these particular disorders in greater detail with the overall goal of elucidating the inextricable role of genetics in the modern practice of oto-rhino-laryngology. Additionally, the experimental methodologies available for gene therapy will be discussed with other emerging technologies. Such research may provide the best chance to eradicate disease at the molecular level, be it down regulating expression of aberrant oncogenes in cancer or replacement of sensory inner hair cells to restore hearing.

References

1 Lejeune J, Gautier M, Turpin R: Etude des chromosomes somatiques de neuf enfants mogoliens. C R Hebd Seances Acad Sci 1959;248:1721–1722.

2 Mullis KB: The unusual origin of the polymerase chain reaction. Sci Am 1990; 262:56–61,64–65.

3 Riordan JR, Rommens JM, Kerem B, Alon N, Rozmahel R, Grzelczak Z, Zielenski J, Lok S, Plavsic N, Chou JL: Identification of the cystic fibrosis gene: cloning and characterization of complementary DNA. Science 1989;245:1066–1073.

4 Evans DG, Huson SM, Donnai D, Neary W, Blair V, Teare D,Newton V, Strachan T, Ramsden R, Harris R: A genetic study of type 2 neurofibromatosis in the United Kingdom. I. Prevalence, mutation rate, fitness, and confirmation of maternal transmission effect on severity. J Med Genet 1992;29:841–846.
5 Friedman LM, Avraham KB: MicroRNAs and epigenetic regulation in the mammalian inner ear: implications for deafness. Mamm Genome 2009;20:581–603.
6 Willems PJ: Genetic causes of hearing loss. NEJM 2000;342:1101–1109.
7 DeStefano AL, Gates GA, Heard-Costa N, Myers RH, Baldwin CT: Genomewide linkage analysis to presbycusis in the Framingham Heart Study. Arch Otolaryngol Head Neck Surg 2003;129: 285–289.
8 Ballana E, Ventayol M, Rabionet R, Gasparini P, Estivill X: Connexins and deafness. URL: http://davinci.crg.es/deafness/, retrieved December 2009.
9 Stevenson VA, Ito M, Milunsky JM: Connexin-30 deletion analysis in Connexin-26 heterozygotes. Genetic Testing 2003;7:151–154.
10 Greinwald JH Jr, Hartnick CJ: The evaluation of children with sensorineural hearing loss. Arch Otolaryngol Head Neck Surg 2002;128:84–87.
11 Lustig LR, Lin D, Venick H, Larky J, Yeagle J, Chinnici J, Polite C, Mhatre AN, Niparko JK, Lalwani AK: GJB2 gene mutations in cochlear implant recipients: prevalence and impact on outcome. Arch Otololaryngol Head Neck Surg 2004;130:541–546.
12 Mäkitie AA, Monni O: Molecular profiling of laryngeal cancer. Expert Rev Anticancer Ther 2009;9:1251–1260.
13 Pérez-Sayáns M, Somoza-Martín JM, Barros-Angueira F, Reboiras-López MD, Gándara Rey JM, García-García A: Genetic and molecular alterations associated with oral squamous cell cancer (review). Oncol Rep 2009;22:1277–1282.
14 Thomas SM, Grandis JR: The current state of head and neck cancer gene therapy. Hum Gene Ther 2009;20:1565–1575.
15 Perez-Ordoñez B, Beauchemin M, Jordan RC: Molecular biology of squamous cell carcinoma of the head and neck. J Clin Pathol. 2006;59:445–453.
16 Pitiyage G, Tilakaratne, Tavassoli M, Warnakulasuriya S: Molecular markers in oral epithelial dysplasia: review. J Oral Pathol Med 2009;38:737–752.
17 Friedman M, Grey P, Venkatesan TK, Bloch I, Chawla P, Caldarelli DD, Coon JS: Prognostic significance of Bcl-2 expression in localized squamous cell carcinoma of the head and neck. Ann Otol Rhinol Laryngol 1997;106:445–450.
18 Zimmermann M, Zouhair A, Azria D, Ozsahin M: The epidermal growth factor receptor (EGFR) in head and neck cancer: its role and treatment implications. Radiat Oncol 2006;1:11.
19 Bikhazi PH, Roeder E, Attaie A, Lalwani AK: Familial paragangliomas: the emerging impact of molecular genetics on evaluation and management. Am J Otol 1999;20:639–643.
20 Patel, NP, Mhatre AN, Lalwani AK: Molecular pathogenesis of skull base tumors. Otol Neurotol 2004;25:636–643.
21 Cole SG, Begbie ME, Wallace GM, Shovlin CL: A new locus for hereditary haemorrhagic telangiectasia (HHT3) maps to chromosome 5. J Med Genet 2005;42:577–582.
22 Marks SC, Kissner DG: Management of sinusitis in adult cystic fibrosis. Am J Rhinol 1997;11:11–14.

Anil K. Lalwani, MD
Department of Otolaryngology, New York University School of Medicine
540 First Avenue, Skirball 7Q
New York, NY 10016 (USA)
Tel. +1 212 263 7167, Fax +1 212 263 2019, E-Mail anil.lalwani@nyumc.org

Alford RL, Sutton VR (eds): Medical Genetics in the Clinical Practice of ORL.
Adv Otorhinolaryngol. Basel, Karger, 2011, vol 70, pp 10–17

Basic Medical Genetics for the Otolaryngologist

Raye L. Alford[a] · Sandra A. Darilek[b]

[a]Bobby R. Alford Department of Otolaryngology – Head and Neck Surgery and [b]Department of Molecular and Human Genetics, Baylor College of Medicine, Houston, Tex., USA

Abstract

Medical genetics is becoming an increasingly important part of the practice of medicine across every medical specialty. For otolaryngologists, understanding the genetic basis of hearing loss, tumors of the head and neck and other otolaryngologic conditions is crucial to effectively incorporating medical genetics information, tools and services into patient care. A clinician who understands the genetic basis of disease, mechanisms of genetic mutation and patterns of inheritance will be positioned to diagnose genetic conditions, interpret genetic test results, assess genetic risks for relatives of patients and refer patients and families for medical genetics and other specialty care. The family medical history is an indispensable tool that, when used properly, can aid in the recognition of genetic susceptibilities within a family and offer opportunities for early intervention. However, obtaining a family medical history is not as simple as it might seem. Knowing what questions to ask, how to properly draw a pedigree and how to recognize patterns of inheritance are critical to obtaining an informative family medical history and using the information in a clinical setting. This article provides a brief introduction to basic medical genetics that includes descriptions of the human genome, the genetic basis of human disease and patterns of inheritance, and a primer for collecting family medical history information.

Basic Medical Genetics

The human genome consists of 46 chromosomes and includes 23 pairs of like chromosomes. Chromosomes 1 through 22 are the autosomal chromosomes. The 23rd pair of chromosomes includes the X and Y and determines sex. The chromosomes are contained within the cell nucleus. Each chromosome is a linear strand of DNA. Genes are discrete segmental sequences of DNA spaced along and embedded within the DNA sequence of the chromosomes.

Chromosomes are inherited through the egg and sperm. An embryo receives one copy of each different chromosome from each parent; that is, one chromosome 1 from dad and one from mom, one chromosome 2 from dad and one from mom, and so on. For the X and Y chromosomes, females can only contribute an X chromosome to an embryo; males can contribute either an X or Y. Genes on the Y chromosome are passed only from fathers to sons.

In females, one X chromosome is inactivated in early development as a mechanism of dosage compensation, although a few genes on the inactive X chromosome escape inactivation. X-inactivation is typically random and females usually have a roughly equal percentage of cells with each of the X chromosomes active, however, significant skewing of X-inactivation can occur and may suggest detrimental mutations involving one X chromosome.

One organelle within the cell, the mitochondrion, also contains DNA. The mitochondrial chromosome is a circular DNA molecule. Each mitochondrion contains several copies of the mitochondrial chromosome and each cell contains many mitochondria. Some mitochondrial proteins are encoded by mitochondrial genes while others are encoded by nuclear genes and imported into the mitochondria. Mitochondria are inherited only through the egg; sperm do not contribute mitochondria to the embryo.

There is a great deal of variability in the human genome. This variability includes: nucleotide substitutions involving only one basepair, called single nucleotide polymorphisms or SNPs, or substitutions involving a few basepairs; insertions, deletions and rearrangements of DNA sequence that can involve any number of nucleotides; changes in length of repetitive DNA sequences; copy number variations involving large stretches of DNA; gross changes in the number or composition of chromosomes. Some DNA sequence variations are associated with medical conditions while others are simply benign variations of no known clinical consequence. Distinguishing between a DNA sequence variation that is a clinically relevant pathogenic mutation and a DNA sequence variation that is a clinically neutral benign polymorphism is crucial for interpreting genetic test results and applying genetic information to patient care.

Patterns of Inheritance

Autosomal Dominant

Autosomal dominant (AD) inheritance is typically observed as the appearance of a condition or trait in every generation of a family. In most cases, individuals affected by autosomal dominant conditions carry a mutation in only one copy of the associated gene. Unless an individual carries two copies of an altered gene for an autosomal dominant condition, each child of an affected individual has a 50% chance of inheriting the affected gene and, except in cases of reduced penetrance, being affected by the condition. Males and females are typically affected with equal frequency and severity unless the condition affects sex-specific organs. Except for cases of new mutations, germline mosaicism or reduced penetrance (which are described later in this article) or cases involving imprinting or anticipation (which will not be described in detail here) unaffected persons do not have affected children.

Autosomal Recessive Inheritance

Autosomal recessive (AR) inheritance is often observed as the appearance of a condition in one generation of a family, i.e. siblings, cousins. However, for common recessive conditions such as Connexin 26-based hearing loss, parent(s) or other relatives may be affected. Autosomal recessive conditions occur when an individual carries mutations in both copies of the associated gene. Unaffected parents of an affected child are typically carriers. Each child of an unaffected carrier couple has a 25% chance of inheriting two affected genes and being affected, a 50% chance of inherited only one affected gene and being an unaffected carrier, and a 25% chance of inheriting two unaffected genes and being an unaffected noncarrier. The risks change if one or both parents are affected; each child of an affected individual will be a carrier and may be affected if the other parent is a carrier or is affected.

Deaf individuals often have children with other deaf individuals, a phenomenon known as assortative mating. In such families, the deafness can appear to be dominantly inherited even though it is not. For example, if two individuals with Connexin 26-related hearing loss have children together all of their children will be affected with hearing loss, even though it is a recessive condition. This is known as pseudodominant inheritance.

X-Linked Inheritance

X-linked inheritance is associated with mutations in genes residing on the X chromosome. Males carrying an X-linked mutation are typically more commonly ascertained and often more severely affected than females carrying an X-linked mutation because males carry only a single X chromosome and therefore lack a functioning copy of the gene. However, females who carry an X-linked mutation may show symptoms of the condition which can range from mild to severe. Further, if there is significantly skewed X-inactivation, females may present with symptoms typical of affected males. Father-to-son transmission of X-linked conditions is never observed because fathers contribute a Y chromosome to their sons. Each child of a female carrying a mutation on one but not both of her X chromosomes has a 50% chance of inheriting the mutation. Each daughter of an affected male will inherit the mutation.

Mitochondrial Inheritance
Mitochondrial inheritance, sometimes described as maternal inheritance, is observed as the occurrence of a condition along the maternal lineage. Mitochondrial inheritance is associated with mutations in genes that reside on the mitochondrial chromosome. It is important to distinguish mitochondrial inheritance from mitochondrial disorders which can be caused by mutations in genes on the autosomal chromosomes as well and thus inherited in an autosomal pattern. Mutations carried on the mitochondrial chromosome are passed from mothers to all of their children; fathers carrying a mitochondrial mutation will not pass the mutation to their children. Mutations carried on the mitochondrial chromosome can be homoplasmic (all mitochondrial chromosomes carry the mutation) or heteroplasmic (only some mitochondrial chromosomes carry the mutation). For heteroplasmic mitochondrial mutations, the severity of the condition in an individual carrying a mutation depends upon the percentage and tissue distribution of mutant mitochondrial chromosomes and can vary considerably even among relatives, complicating prediction of phenotype and genetic counseling.

Multifactorial Conditions
Multifactorial conditions result from the interaction of genetic and environmental factors. Risk estimates for relatives of affected individuals are typically empiric and based on data from population studies. When estimating risks for relatives of an affected individual, one must consider the degree of relatedness between the at-risk individual and the affected individual, i.e. first-degree relatives typically have higher risks than third-degree relatives.

Genetic Phenomena that Impact Assessment of Patterns of Inheritance

New Mutations
Genetic mutations that occur during gametogenesis or very early after fertilization are present in an affected child but not in either parent. The time during development at which a new mutation occurs affects the tissue distribution of the mutation (mosaicism), the symptomatic expression of the condition, and the risks for future offspring. Genetic conditions caused by new mutations are typically dominant conditions, where a mutation in only one copy of a gene is sufficient to cause the condition, or X-linked or mitochondrial conditions. In pedigrees, new mutations are observed as sporadic occurrence of a genetic condition, without a family history of the condition. For X-linked conditions, it is often the mothers of affected sons who carry the new mutation. This is important to recognize because a carrier mother is at risk for having additional affected sons and carrier daughters. For some genetic conditions, particularly those caused by point mutations, an advanced paternal age effect is seen where the likelihood of having an affected child increases with paternal age.

Mosaicism: Germline and Somatic
When a new mutation occurs after fertilization, some but not all the cells of the individual carry

the mutation: this is called mosaicism. When mosaicism involves only egg or sperm cells, or their precursors, it is called germline mosaicism. When mosaicism involves two or more tissues in the body, one of which may or may not be germline, it is called somatic mosaicism. The degree of mosaicism in an individual can impact clinical presentation of the condition and recurrence risk. When the germline is involved, there is a risk that offspring of the mosaic individual might be affected by the condition. Because assessment of germline mosaicism is not presently possible, genetic risk estimates for conditions with documented germline mosaicism are empiric and based on population data.

Reduced Penetrance

Penetrance is an on/off state: individuals carrying mutations in a gene either show signs of the condition or they do not. When some but not all of the individuals in a population who carry mutations in a particular gene show signs of the associated condition, the condition is said to demonstrate reduced penetrance. Not all genetic conditions demonstrate reduced penetrance; however, for some, it is characteristic of the condition. Knowing whether a particular genetic condition demonstrates reduced penetrance is important for estimating the likelihood that an individual who inherits a mutation in the associated gene will develop the condition. It is important to be aware that some or all phenotypic features of a condition may not appear early in life but rather may develop with age. In addition, for some conditions, phenotypic features can be quite subtle and a focused physical exam or diagnostic evaluation might reveal features not previously evident to the individual or their health care providers.

Variable Expressivity

Variable expressivity, or variability, is a like a dial: individuals carrying mutations in a gene show variation in the clinical expression of the associated condition. Some individuals may show only a few signs of a condition while others may show more; some individuals may experience mild symptoms while others' symptoms are more debilitating; some individuals may have slow progression while others experience a more rapid or aggressive course of the condition. Variable expressivity can be interfamilial (between unrelated families) and/or intrafamilial (between relatives within a family) and can complicate diagnosis of a condition, especially if the symptoms can be subtle enough to be missed in relatives or nonspecific enough to be suggestive of several different diagnoses. Strictly speaking, virtually every genetic condition demonstrates some degree of inter-individual variability. However, for some conditions, variability is particularly noteworthy because it impacts detection and diagnosis and prediction of phenotype and genetic risk for relatives of an affected individual.

Genetic Heterogeneity

There are two types of genetic heterogeneity: allelic and locus. Allelic heterogeneity occurs when different mutations within a single gene cause a condition. Locus heterogeneity occurs when one or more mutations in different genes cause a condition. Genetic heterogeneity impacts genetic testing methodologies, prediction of prognosis and genetic counseling. Genetic tests for conditions with genetic heterogeneity that employ methods capable of detecting only one or a few mutations associated with a condition may miss some mutations and return negative results when a patient, in fact, carries a mutation that was not detected by the test. Further, understanding whether a mutation is associated with mild or severe symptoms or slow or rapid disease progression is important for estimating prognosis and establishing a therapeutic plan. Finally, knowing that a condition can be inherited in a variety of patterns, i.e. autosomal dominant, autosomal recessive and/or X-linked, is crucial for interpreting family medical history information and providing accurate genetic counseling.

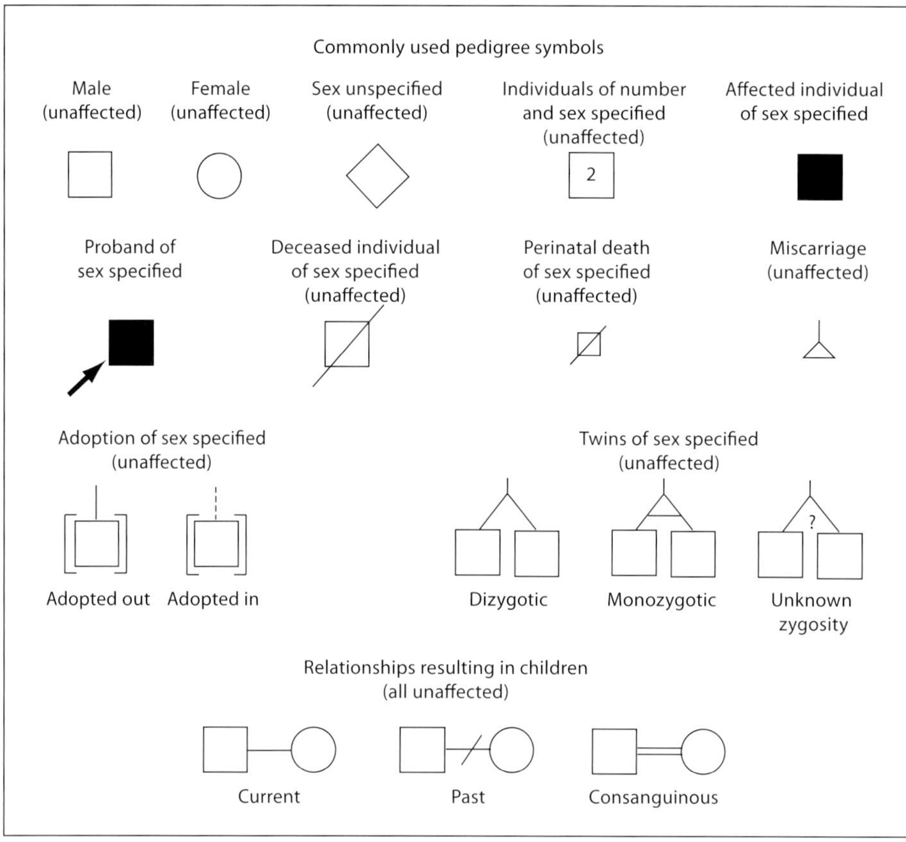

Fig. 1. Commonly used pedigree symbols.

For further reading on concepts in medical genetics see Thompson & Thompson Genetics in Medicine [1].

Obtaining a Family Medical History in the Otolaryngology Clinic

Obtaining a thorough family medical history, or family history, can provide valuable information to assist in determining, for example, the etiology of hearing loss in a patient or whether a neoplasia of the head and neck might be part of a larger genetic syndrome or familial predisposition to cancer. Analysis of the family history can also aid in making a specific diagnosis or determining the most appropriate tests to order and can reveal the inheritance pattern of a condition in a family and offer information about the natural history of the condition.

The simplest way to document a family history is by drawing a pedigree. Figure 1 contains the basic symbols used to construct a pedigree. Typically, a three-generation pedigree is constructed by first obtaining information on the patient, and then moving on to the patient's first-degree relatives (parents, children, and siblings), second-degree relatives (half-siblings, grandparents, aunts and uncles, nieces and nephews, and grandchildren) and third-degree relatives (first cousins), obtaining information about both maternal and paternal family members. It is important to ascertain whether all siblings within a sibship have the same parents and whether all children were conceived with the same partner and to indicate these relationships on the pedigree. Many patients will not mention that siblings are actually half-siblings or that their children have different fathers/mothers without specifically being asked and this information can impact evaluation of a pedigree.

For each individual in the pedigree, the following information can be important: current age, physical and mental health status, or age at death and cause of death. For individuals affected with a particular condition, it is important, if known, to note the age at onset or age at diagnosis and to be as specific and accurate about the diagnosis as possible. For example, with respect to hearing loss it is important to note if the hearing loss is congenital or was noted later, progressive or non-progressive, unilateral or bilateral, and conductive, sensorineural, or mixed. If a specific etiology for a condition is known, that information can be noted and if genetic testing has been performed the results can be included (e.g. note *GJB2*- [Connexin 26-] related hearing loss; homozygous c.35delG mutation or c.35delG/c.35delG for Connexin 26-related hearing loss due to the presence of two copies of the c.35delG mutation determined by genetic testing). Information recorded on the pedigree will need to be concise; however, the use of multiple abbreviations can become confusing. It is helpful to make note of and define any abbreviations or short-hand used in the pedigree in a key. Two other pieces of information are also of particular interest in a pedigree: ethnicity and consanguinity. The ethnic background of the family, both the maternal and paternal sides, can be particularly important as some genetic conditions are more common in specific ethnic backgrounds. When obtaining this information, it is often most useful to ask about the family's country of origin and if they belong to a particular ethnic group from within that country (e.g. Ashkenazi Jews from Eastern Europe and Russia or Sephardic Jews from the Mediterranean). Also important to note is whether any family members are related to one another, particularly the parents of the individual being evaluated. If consanguinity is noted, the exact nature of the consanguinity (first cousins, second cousins, first cousins once-removed, etc.) and which relatives are shared can be indicated. A sample three-generation pedigree is shown in figure 2 for a family segregating hearing loss. Note how the hearing loss in this family appears to be inherited in an autosomal dominant manner, however, genetic testing reveals this family is segregating the most common form of autosomal recessive nonsyndromic sensorineural hearing loss caused by mutations in the *GJB2* gene encoding the protein Connexin 26. As discussed previously, this phenomenon, known as pseudodominant inheritance, can be observed when there is a high carrier frequency of the condition in the population.

When the pedigree appears complete, a series of general and targeted questions can also be asked. This may seem redundant but often patients will recall additional information after completion of the pedigree when asked specific questions. General questions can include whether there is any family history of mental retardation, birth defects, inherited conditions, multiple miscarriages, infant deaths or stillbirths, or early-onset cancer. Targeted questions can provide further clues to narrow down a differential diagnosis. For example, when taking a family history focused on hearing loss, the following conditions are of particular interest:

1 Visual anomalies – iris heterochromia, ocular malformation, retinitis pigmentosa, vision loss, night blindness, moderate-severe myopia, retinal detachment, early cataracts, congenital glaucoma, optic atrophy.
2 Facial/cervical dysmorphology – synophrys, dystopia canthorum, abnormal ear shape or size, preauricular pits, aural atresia, branchial cysts or fistulas, cleft lip and/or palate, dental anomalies, micrognathia.

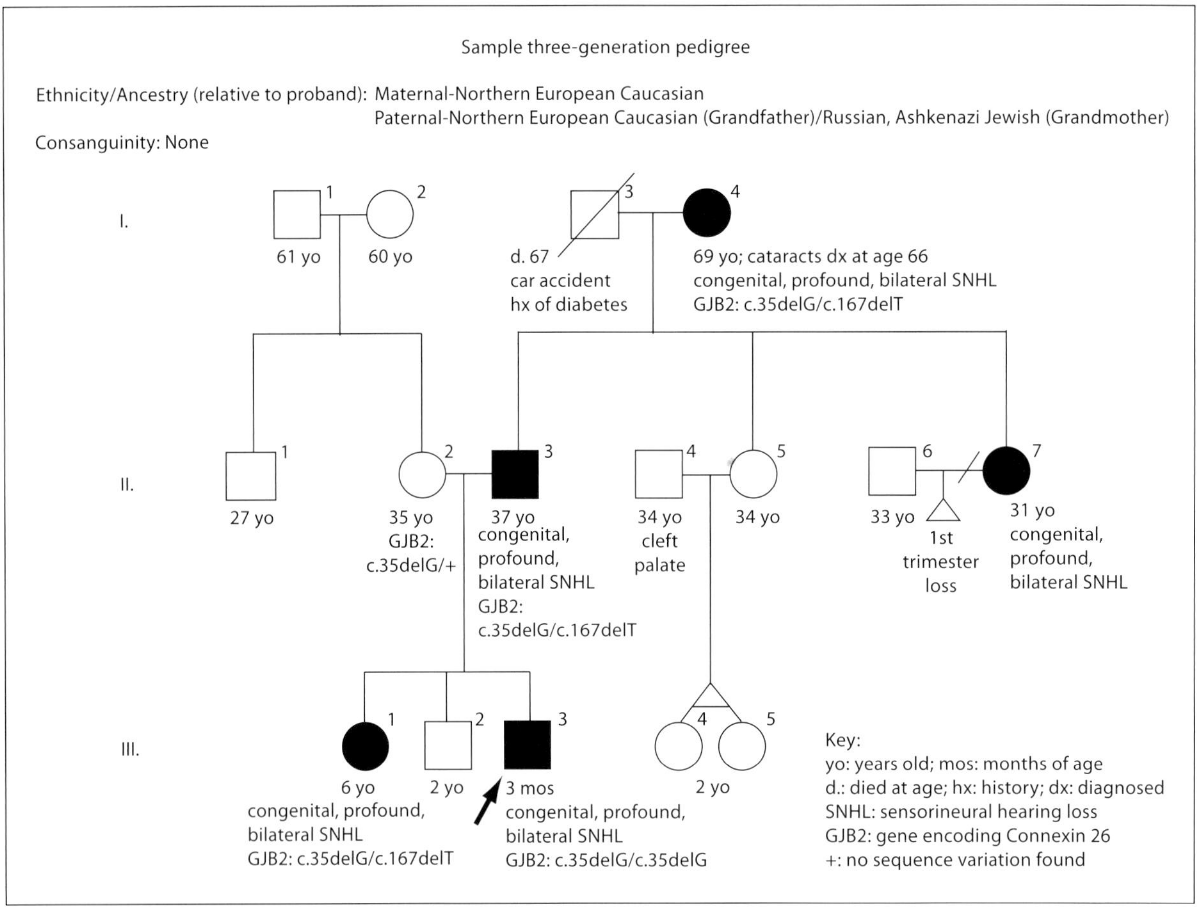

Fig. 2. Three-generation pedigree. A sample three-generation pedigree is shown for a family segregating hearing loss. Although not frequently used in clinical pedigrees, the numbering of generations and individuals is used when discussion of individuals is required and anonymity needs to be preserved, such as publications and presentations. Individual III-3 is the proband. Individuals I-4, II-7 and III-1 are affected females; individuals II-3 and III-3 are affected males. Individuals I-2, II-2, II-5, III-4 and III-5 are unaffected females; individuals I-1, I-3, II-1, II-4, II-6 and III-2 are unaffected males. III-4 and III-5 are monozygotic twin girls. I-3 is deceased. II-6 and II-7 are divorced; together, they had one miscarriage.

3 Endocrine abnormalities – thyromegaly, diabetes, hypothyroidism.
4 Cardiac signs or symptoms – syncope, sudden death, arrhythmia, prolonged QT interval, fainting spells, congenital heart defect.
5 Renal abnormalities – hematuria, proteinuria, structural renal defects.
6 Integumentary changes – premature graying, white forelock, abnormal pigmentation, dry skin/keratoderma.

When focusing on hereditary neoplasias of the head and neck, the following tumors are of particular interest: parathyroid tumors, pituitary tumors, medullary thyroid tumors, pheochromocytomas, vestibular schwannomas, and paragangliomas. If the age at diagnosis for any affected individual is known, that information can also be noted.

The importance of the family medical history as a tool for ascertaining genetic conditions cannot be underestimated. Accuracy and detail are of paramount importance. This simple task can provide information useful for determining the etiology of a condition and illuminate valuable clues that can make the process of obtaining a specific diagnosis more efficient.

For further reading on principles of genetic counseling see Standardized Human Pedigree Nomenclature: Update and Assessment of the Recommendations of the National Society of Genetic Counselors [2], A Guide to Genetic Counseling [3] and Practical Genetic Counselling [4].

Resources

American College of Medical Genetics. www.acmg.net
National Society of Genetic Counselors. www.nsgc.org
Family Health History Tool From The Genetic Alliance: www.doesitruninthefamily.org
My Family Health Portrait tool from the US Surgeon General:
https://familyhistory.hhs.gov/fhh-web/home.action
Know Your Family Health History Campaign of the American Society of Human Genetics and The Genetic Alliance: www.talkhealthhistory.org
GeneClinics – GeneTests – GeneReviews. www.genetests.org
Genetics Home Reference. http://ghr.nlm.nih.gov/
Online Mendelian Inheritance in Man (OMIM). www.ncbi.nlm.nih.gov/omim/
ACMG Basics: Genetics for Providers. An Educational CME Activity. www.acmg.net.

References

1 Nussbaum RL, McInnes RR, Willard HF: Thompson & Thompson Genetics in Medicine, ed 7. Philadelphia, Saunders/Elsevier, 2007.

2 Bennett RL, French KS, Resta RG, Doyle DL: Standardized human pedigree nomenclature: update and assessment of the recommendations of the National Society of Genetic Counselors. J Genet Couns 2008;17:424–433.

3 Baker DL, Schuette JL, Uhlmann WR (eds): A Guide to Genetic Counseling. New York, Wiley-Liss, 1998.

4 Harper PS: Practical Genetic Counselling, ed 6. London, Arnold, 2004.

Raye L. Alford, PhD, FACMG
Bobby R. Alford Department of Otolaryngology – Head and Neck Surgery
Baylor College of Medicine, One Baylor Plaza, NA102
Houston, TX 77030 (USA)
Tel. +1 713 798 8599, Fax +1 713 798 3403, E-Mail ralford@bcm.edu

Alford RL, Sutton VR (eds): Medical Genetics in the Clinical Practice of ORL.
Adv Otorhinolaryngol. Basel, Karger, 2011, vol 70, pp 18–24

Ordering Genetic Tests and Interpreting the Results

Joshua L. Deignan · Wayne W. Grody

University of California Los Angeles, Los Angeles, Calif., USA

Abstract

As the number of clinical genetic laboratories becomes more abundant, it will become increasingly challenging for clinicians in the medical and surgical specialties to navigate the vast menus of testing available and decide upon the most appropriate approach for molecular diagnosis of a particular disorder. There are many associated ethical and psychosocial issues involved with ordering clinical genetic tests of which practitioners need to remain aware, including predictive testing of minors, implications of the test result for other family members, theoretical risks of insurance or employment discrimination, and how to appropriately counsel families once test results have been finalized and reported. Finally, as the field of genetic testing changes so rapidly, it will be of great help for otolaryngologists to familiarize themselves and remain up to date with the general terminology and interpretive criteria that go into clinical molecular genetic laboratory reports, in order to make it useful and understandable to clinicians and patients.

Choosing a Laboratory

For otolaryngologic disorders requiring more than a clinical diagnosis, molecular diagnostic testing is often required. For relatively common genetic disorders such as cystic fibrosis, there is an abundance of clinical laboratories that offer relevant and widely accepted testing, but for other more rare disorders, the selection of capable clinical laboratories and knowledgeable directors may be more limited. In the absence of any prior experience or personal knowledge of a clinical laboratory performing the specific test for a disorder which one is trying to diagnose, GeneTests (http://www.genetests.org) [1] is likely the best place to start.

GeneTests provides a wealth of information on many genetic disorders and includes a clinical description of the disorder as well as the mode(s) of inheritance, the most appropriate testing strategies, genetic counseling recommendations, clinical management, and differential diagnosis to help rule out other genetic or acquired conditions with overlapping phenotypes. Furthermore, GeneTests is an easy route for assessing clinical test availability either by disease, gene name, or location. It offers both names and contact information for clinical laboratories performing testing as well as the type of testing being offered. For example, a search for the prominent otologic disorder neurofibromatosis type 2 (website accessed on January 21, 2010) reveals that there are 13 laboratories that offer testing, the majority of which offer full-gene sequencing, deletion/duplication analysis, or both. An individual laboratory can then be contacted using the telephone numbers or e-mail addresses provided for more specific information about other details such as test methodology, pricing, sample requirements, and turnaround time.

Referring physicians should make sure that the laboratory chosen is appropriately adhering to standard regulatory and quality assurance guidelines in the field. At the very least, the lab should be licensed under the Clinical Laboratory Improvement Amendments (CLIA) and accredited by the College of American Pathologists. Conveniently, all laboratories listed in the GeneTests database are required to provide evidence of their current accreditation and its expiration date. However, some extremely rare genetic diseases may only be performed in one or two laboratories in the world, and sometimes these are research, not clinical, laboratories. This will be clearly stated in GeneTests and it must be recognized that any specimen sent to such laboratories will be tested on a research basis. In the absence of any available testing in a CLIA-certified lab, it may be necessary to proceed this way, but the ordering physician should be aware that, strictly speaking, research laboratories are not supposed to give out test result information for use in medical management.

Choosing the Right Test

Once a list of clinical laboratories offering testing for a particular disorder is obtained, trying to decipher the most appropriate test and navigate through the various methodologies becomes the next hurdle. The most common methodology for disorders in which a specific disease-causing mutation or set of mutations is unknown is DNA sequencing (also called Sanger sequencing after the person who first developed the method). With this method, a region of interest (usually a single exon or coding region of a gene, or all the exons) is amplified and then subjected to a secondary sequencing reaction, resulting in a series of products which can be read on a genetic analyzer (made by Applied Biosystems, Foster City, Calif., USA). This allows visualization of the nucleotide that exists at each position in the exon through the use of fluorescent tags. If the instrument detects that two different nucleotides are present at a specific location (as in the case of a heterozygous germline mutation), signals for the fluorescent tags from both nucleotides will appear. For example, several of the laboratories which perform testing for neurofibromatosis type 2 perform sequencing of all coding exons (1–17) as their test method of choice. This will theoretically pick up the greatest number of possible mutations, wherever they may lie within the gene, provided they do not fall within introns or other noncoding regions which are usually not sequenced.

In addition to providing information about test methodology, GeneTests also provides contact information for genetic counselors employed by the genetic diagnostic laboratory that are capable of discussing testing algorithms, test logistics and particular clinical situations with a patient or physician by phone or e-mail. Genetic counselors are masters-level members of the medical genetics team. While they may not be familiar to many practicing otorhinolaryngologists, they represent a valuable resource and convenient point of entry into the genetic testing milieu. A preliminary conversation with one of them can help sort out which particular test is the most appropriate for a specific clinical situation, or even whether genetic testing is warranted at all. Otorhinolaryngologists based at larger institutions may be able to access a genetic counselor in-house, typically associated with either the Pediatrics or Obstetrics departments. Those in smaller practices can avail themselves of the genetic counselors employed by the larger genetic testing laboratories to which the patient specimen will likely be sent.

Issues Related to Testing Minors

As stated in the 1995 ASHG/ACMG report on Genetic Testing in Children and Adolescents [2], when considering genetic testing on minors it is important to advocate on behalf of the child while simultaneously weighing the medical and social harms and benefits of the testing. This notion was further codified by the NIH/DOE Task Force on Genetic Testing [3], which cautioned that children should not undergo predictive testing for adult-onset disorders unless there is some preventive medical intervention available that would be lost if the testing was deferred to adulthood. For example, in a completely penetrant, adult-onset condition such as Huntington disease where no symptoms typically manifest until around age 35, performing testing on a child should be discouraged since there is no harm in waiting until they are of legal adult age and can make an informed decision about whether they want to be tested. However, for an autosomal-dominant disorder such as multiple endocrine neoplasia type 2 in which serious neoplasias of the head and neck region, such as medullary carcinoma of the thyroid, can begin to manifest at a very early age, diagnostic testing of suspected cases or at-risk individuals (even at a young age) is warranted. This is because there are various screening and surgical interventions that may improve prognosis, and diagnosis through genetic testing for mutations in the *RET* gene may be required in order to proceed with these interventions. Another example is familial adenomatous polyposis and the related Gardner syndrome, in which jaw osteomas and other head and neck lesions may be a feature and the more threatening colon polyps may begin to appear in childhood; in such children at risk (i.e. offspring of an affected parent), it is recommended that testing for mutations in the *APC* gene be performed by about age 10. In contrast, for symptomatic conditions such as CHARGE syndrome and Usher syndrome (types I and II), where the diagnosis is already suspected based on clinical grounds, confirmatory molecular genetic testing on minors is also reasonable, as no further harm can result from performing the testing, and the child and family will all benefit by the arrival at a definitive diagnosis. That diagnosis will also reveal the mode of inheritance (dominant, recessive, or X-linked), which can enable accurate risk assessment for recurrence in future children of the patient's parents.

Informed Consent

Otorhinolaryngologists are of course familiar with informed consent procedures prior to surgery, but the notion of obtaining specific informed consent for a diagnostic laboratory test, especially one performed on a simple blood specimen, may seem somewhat foreign. Because of the rather checkered history of genetic testing, various eugenics movements in the United States and elsewhere, and the race/ethnicity abuses of Nazi Germany, a tradition has developed in some quarters for obtaining informed consent for genetic testing, and has become mandated in some jurisdictions such as New York State. However, the need for doing so is by no means broadly agreed upon, even within the medical genetics community. The NIH/DOE Task Force, among many other groups, has wrestled with this controversy, and issued a compromise recommendation [3]: namely, that pre-test informed consent should be obtained for predictive (i.e. presymptomatic) genetic tests such as Hungtington disease and familial breast/ovarian cancer (BRCA1 and BRCA2 gene mutations), but should not be required for diagnostic testing in an already-symptomatic patient. The rationale behind this is that predictive testing in a healthy individual carries a significant psychosocial risk, whereas genetic testing to confirm a diagnosis in a symptomatic individual falls squarely within the diagnostic work-up of the patient's problem, which would be covered by the consent for treatment, which has presumably already been obtained.

Nevertheless, some referral laboratories to which the patient's specimen may be sent may, depending on their own local protocols, request evidence of informed consent. Often this will be in the form of a simple check-box or signature line on the laboratory requisition form, where the ordering physician can attest to the fact that some sort of pre-test counseling and informed consent was administered. Other laboratories may actually have and provide their own customized informed consent form which will need to be read and signed by the patient and must accompany the specimen when it is sent to the laboratory.

GINA

On May 21, 2008, President George W. Bush signed into law the Genetic Information Nondiscrimination Act (GINA) that protects Americans against discrimination based on their genetic information when it involves health insurance and employment. The regulations for Title I (which became effective on December 7, 2009) prohibit insurance companies from using genetic information to discriminate against insured individuals and forbid them from requiring individuals to provide genetic information to the insurers. Genetic information also cannot be used as a pre-existing condition. The final regulations for Title II of GINA (which prohibits employee discrimination based on genetic information) have not yet been issued.

As an example, an individual with neurofibromatosis type 2 (NF2) is expected to develop bilateral vestibular schwannomas by age 30 which often require surgery. As NF2 is a completely penetrant autosomal-dominant disorder and half of the affected individuals have an affected parent with the same disorder, prior knowledge about their genetic predisposition to developing schwannomas was previously thought to be a liability for the purposes of health insurance. However, after the passage of GINA, even if an individual was tested early on in childhood and was confirmed to have inherited a known disease-causing variant for NF2 from their affected parent, this information could not be used to deny payment of necessary surgical treatments by the insurance company. Theoretically, at least, this law should remove some of the potential stigma of positive genetic test results and should reduce the apprehension many patients may have in approaching such testing. However, its effectiveness in practice has yet to be tested [4].

What Genetic Tests Can Reveal About Relatives

DNA variants can be either inherited from an affected parent or arise de novo in a child, meaning the proband (affected individual) is the first one in the pedigree whose genome contains a specific variation. Both scenarios have important implications that need to be taken into consideration when evaluating the results of genetic testing. For the parents of an individual affected with an autosomal-dominant disorder (such as NF2), a lack of phenotype in the parents is most often due to a de novo mutation in the proband or a case of either reduced penetrance or mosaicism in a parent (a mixture of normal and mutant-containing cells) resulting in an absent or mild phenotype. However, a lack of phenotype in the parents of an individual with an autosomal-recessive disorder (such as nonsyndromic sensorineural hereditary hearing loss caused by mutations in the connexin-26 [*GJB2*] gene) reveals nothing about the genetic status of the parents. It is much more likely that each parent is a carrier for one mutation than it would be for the proband to have developed two disease-causing mutations de novo in order to develop the disorder, so the carrier status of the parents is usually inferred by the finding of an individual affected by an autosomal recessive disorder, and they are counseled that there is a likely 25% recurrence risk with each subsequent pregnancy. Actual DNA testing of the parents will confirm the existence and identity of their carrier mutations and allow for prenatal testing in a future pregnancy.

Whether the proband has an autosomal-recessive or autosomal-dominant disorder also provides information about the siblings. In the case of a connexin-26-positive individual, a sibling would be expected to have a 25% chance of being affected with the disorder, a 50% chance of being a carrier, and a 25% chance of having inherited no disease-causing variants. In the case of inherited NF2, a sibling would be expected to have a 50% chance of being affected with the disorder and a 50% chance of being unaffected. However, if it is a true *de novo* case, a sibling should not be affected or at risk unless mosaicism is present in one of the parents.

What Positive and Negative Test Results Mean

In genetic testing, as in most clinical laboratory testing, an individual would usually prefer to receive a 'negative' result. Negative results typically indicate that the genetic alteration or alterations in question were not found, and the DNA sequence at that particular location in the patient is 'normal' (or, more specifically, that it matches the sequence which is considered to be present in the majority of individuals who do not exhibit symptoms of the particular disorder). On the other hand, a positive result means that a genetic alteration was found. It can involve a single nucleotide or series of nucleotide bases, it can change an amino acid in the protein product of the gene (missense mutation), it can leave the amino acid unaltered (polymorphism or silent mutation), it can cause termination (premature truncation) of the protein (nonsense mutation), it can add extra nucleotides to the DNA sequence (insertion), and it can eliminate nucleotides from the DNA sequence (deletion). Whatever type of alteration exists, it must always be analyzed in the context of its effect on the protein, which is usually the most important functional element dictated by the genetic code.

In the case of connexin-26 deafness, the majority of the genetic changes are frameshift mutations which eliminate a G (guanidine) nucleotide 35 bases from the start of the protein-coding sequence. This mutation is designated as c.35delG, and its effect is that the entire downstream protein-coding sequence is shifted by one base. Since each set of three bases codes for one amino acid, and multiple amino acids comprise a protein, the protein is now made incorrectly.

Mutations, Polymorphisms, and Variants of Unknown Significance

So what constitutes a true mutation? A mutation should have an established clinical correlation with multiple studies having been done to determine that it is in fact responsible for causing or contributing significantly to the disorder. If this is true, it should not be found in individuals without biological manifestations of the disorder, although it is possible to have a known mutation in an individual without any symptoms (either due to reduced penetrance or carrier status for a recessive disease). On the other hand, the definition of a polymorphism is any benign genetic variant that is present in greater than 1% of the general population. These are expected to be benign (not disease-causing) and are variable between individuals much like a given person's last name; individuals are expected to have different last names if they are unrelated, but two unrelated individuals can still have the same last name by chance. Similarly, two unrelated individuals may or may not have the same sequence present at a given polymorphic site, but if they differ it is likely just due to normal variation in the population.

Variants of unknown significance (or VUSs as they are typically known) can be a more perplexing story and present a real challenge in clinical interpretation, genetic counseling, and management. Most often, these are missense mutations (alteration of an amino acid) with no published or otherwise documented association with disease or with conflicting associations in the literature.

Nonsense mutations are typically not VUSs, as their effect on protein termination is so severe that by definition they can be used to justify the phenotype if the disorder is known to be due to a failure of protein function. In an autosomal recessive disorder like Pendred syndrome, where three common mutations in the *SLC26A4* gene exist in persons of northern European descent (p.L236P, p.T416P, c.1001 + 1G>A), complete sequencing of the gene in a patient may reveal one of these mutations as well as another missense mutation that has never been reported before. It is typically up to the laboratory director to make the determination as to whether a particular DNA variant likely represents a true mutation or is simply a polymorphism using all resources available [5]. However, sometimes this is simply not possible, and the patient and physician are left with as big a question mark hanging over them after the testing as was there before the test. In such cases it is often helpful for the clinician to contact the laboratory director to discuss the patient's phenotype, medical and family history to gain a better understanding of the laboratory results.

Evolving Knowledge and Technology and the Importance of Follow-Up

One of the most important and challenging duties for those who choose to offer clinical genetic testing is to remain up-to-date. What was known yesterday about a particular condition may not be true today, and what is true today may not be true tomorrow. The clinical genetics laboratory director has the responsibility to not only provide clinicians with the answers to a question (the analytic test results) but also to give them a clear explanation of what those results actually mean (the clinical utility); this is necessary in order to guide how to proceed in treating or managing the patient. As an example, the status of VUSs are constantly being updated and revised based on testing of larger populations, so databases of mutations require constant revision. Finally, technological platforms change at an alarming rate, so that which was undetectable yesterday may be detectable today, and it is the job of the clinical laboratory to determine if that has any meaning for better answering a clinician's question. On the other hand, it is understood that these laboratories do not have the resources to follow-up all patients tested after an interim of many years, and the so-called 'duty to re-contact' has been left more to the ordering physicians or to the patients themselves (who must assume some responsibility in keeping current with new developments related to their disease) [6]. This is yet one more reason why it is so important for otorhinolaryngologists and all other non-genetic specialists to remain facile with this technology in this age of molecular medicine.

There is plenty of ancillary support and sources of information for those who need it and for patients whose situation warrants a genetics referral. Genetic counselors are available in any institution that offers medical genetics, cancer genetics, or prenatal genetics services, as well as at most genetic testing laboratories. They represent an excellent entry into the world of genetic medicine and can put the referring physician in touch with an MD medical geneticist as needed. The medical genetics consultation is most helpful in assessing genetic risk, appropriateness of testing, interpretation of complex genetic test results, and generally integrating disparate clinical and laboratory findings across various body systems (since the discipline spans essentially all other medical specialties). In addition, there are numerous online resources available to help point the non-genetic specialist in the right direction. A good place to start is the GeneTests/GeneClinics website [www.genetests.org], which provides a directory of genetic testing laboratories for all available diseases, clinical and scientific background on the diseases tested, along with a directory of genetics clinics in all geographic areas. Further referral information can be found on the organization websites of the American College of Medical Genetics [www.acmg.net] and the National Society of Genetic Counselors [www.nsgc.org]. No otorhinolaryngologist should feel at a loss for ordering and understanding genetic tests with the help of these resources.

References

1 GeneTests: Medical Genetics Information Resource (database online). Copyright, University of Washington, Seattle, 1993–2010. Available at http://www.genetests.org.

2 American Society of Human Genetics Board of Directors, American College of Medical Genetics Board of Directors: Points to consider: ethical, legal, and psychosocial implications of genetic testing in children and adolescents. Am J Hum Genet 1995;57:1233–1241.

3 Holtzman N, Murphy P, Watson M, Barr P: Predictive genetic testing: from basic research to clinical practice. Science 1997;278:602–605.

4 Erwin C: Legal update: living with the Genetic Information Nondiscrimination Act. Genet Med 2008;10:869–873.

5 Richards CS, Bale S, Bellissimo DB, Das S, Grody WW, Hegde MR, Lyon E, Ward BE, Molecular Subcommittee of the ACMG Laboratory Quality Assurance Committee: ACMG recommendations for standards for interpretation and reporting of sequence variations: revisions 2007. Genet Med 2008;10:294–300.

6 American College of Medical Genetics, Social Ethical and Legal Issues Committee: Duty to recontact. Genet Med 1999;1:171–172.

Wayne W. Grody, MD, PhD
Departments of Pathology and Laboratory Medicine and Pediatrics
UCLA School of Medicine, 10833 Le Conte Ave.
Los Angeles, CA 90095–1732 (USA)
Tel. +1 310 825 5648, Fax +1 310 794 4840, E-Mail wgrody@mednet.ucla.edu

Alford RL, Sutton VR (eds): Medical Genetics in the Clinical Practice of ORL.
Adv Otorhinolaryngol. Basel, Karger, 2011, vol 70, pp 25–27

Referring Patients for a Medical Genetics Consultation and Genetic Counseling

V. Reid Sutton

Department of Molecular and Human Genetics, Baylor College of Medicine and Texas Children's Hospital, Houston, Tex., USA

Abstract

Clinical geneticists and genetic counselors provide diagnosis and counseling for genetic disorders affecting every organ system and every age group. Genetic counselors are more focused on informing patients and families about the inheritance of a genetic disorder and providing recurrence risk counseling, support and information about a diagnosis and reproductive options. Medical geneticists may also share some of these roles in addition to establishing a diagnosis and providing medical management. Medical Geneticists receive training in ACGME-accredited residency programs and are certified by the American Board of Medical Genetics. Genetic counseling is a masters degree program and certification is granted by the American Board of Genetic Counseling. When a patient/family is referred to a Clinical Geneticist, they may expect a thorough evaluation in an effort to establish a diagnosis that may provide information about etiology, prognosis, therapy and recurrence risk.

Scope of Practice of Clinical Genetics

The specialty of medical genetics encompasses all age ranges and a broad variety of patients. Individuals and couples may seek out a geneticist or genetic counselor for prenatal evaluation, and while pediatric patients make up the bulk of most clinical geneticists' practices, adults may also be referred for evaluation. Some Clinical Geneticists restrict their practice to a specific age range or disease group, while others may see a very wide variety of ages and disorders. Common groups of diseases seen and the roles of the geneticist may include:

- Preconception evaluation and counseling including genetic risk assessment for relatives of affected individuals.
- Prenatal evaluation and counseling.
- Diagnostic evaluation of individuals with single or multiple congenital anomalies.
- Diagnosis and management of individuals with genetic syndromes and chromosome abnormalities.
- Diagnosis and dietary and medical management of inborn errors of metabolism (e.g. urea cycle disorders, organic acidemias).
- Medical management and enzyme replacement therapy for lysosomal storage disorders (e.g. Gaucher, Fabry, Hurler diseases).
- Diagnosis and management of connective tissue disorders (e.g. Marfan, Ehlers-Danlos syndromes).
- Diagnosis and counseling for cancer genetic syndromes (e.g. multiple endocrine neoplasia syndromes).
- Diagnosis and continuing care for neurofibromatosis and tuberous sclerosis.

- Diagnosis and treatment of osteogenesis imperfecta (brittle bone disease) and other skeletal dysplasias.
- Diagnosis and care for adults presenting with genetic disorders (e.g. hereditary hemorrhagic telangectasia, Osler-Weber-Rendu, Charcot-Marie-Tooth disease).

Qualifications and Training of a Medical Geneticist

The American Board of Medical Genetics was founded in 1980, is a member of the American Board of Medical Specialties and currently administers a certifying examination every 2 years, in conjunction with the National Board of Medical Examiners. In order to be a candidate for board certification in medical genetics, in the United States, a physician must complete at least 2 years of residency in an ACGME-accredited residency program as well as 2 years of training in an ACGME-accredited medical genetics residency. The training and certification process in Canada is similar to the United States. In Western Europe, there is training in clinical genetics; however, board certification in medical genetics is not available in all countries. Current information about the status of genetic residency training and board certification in Europe can be found on the website of the European Society of Human Genetics (www.eshg.org). Most geneticists in the United States are required to participate in the American Board of Medical Genetics maintenance of certification program.

Qualifications and Training of a Genetic Counselor

Training in genetic counseling involves graduate-level coursework in human genetics, genetic principals and counseling skills. Those who successfully complete a training program receive a master's degree in genetic counseling and are eligible for board certification through the American Board of Genetic Counseling. The certifying examination is given every 2 years and those certified after 1996 are required to participate in the recertification program.

When to Refer to a Medical Geneticist

A full listing of indications for genetic referral can be found in a practice guideline located on the website of the American College of Medical Genetics (http://www.acmg.net/AM/Template.cfm?-Section = Practice_Guidelines&Template = /CM/ContentDisplay.cfm&ContentID = 2748) [1]. The more common reasons an otolaryngologist might refer a patient to a medical geneticist include:

- Sensorineural hearing loss.
- Cleft lip and/or cleft palate.
- Multiple birth defects.
- Acoustic neuroma.
- Telangectasias of the nasal mucosa.
- Cancers of the head and neck that may be associated with a cancer genetic syndrome or hereditary predisposition to cancer.

The otolaryngologist may expect that the geneticist will perform a diagnostic evaluation, order and interpret diagnostic studies, when needed, counsel the individual/family about prognosis and recurrence risk and manage medical care, when indicated (e.g. recommended medical care and surveillance for hereditary hemorrhagic telangectasia and neurofibromatosis type 2, multiple endocrine neoplasia syndromes and hereditary paraganglioma).

When to Refer to a Genetic Counselor

Patients or families who would like information about inheritance and recurrence risk of a particular condition should be referred to a genetic counselor.

Elements of a Genetic Evaluation

Medical Geneticist

- Detailed medical/surgical history.
- 3–4 generations pedigree.
- Physical examination.
- Order diagnostic tests.
- Provide information about prognosis and recurrence risk.
- Provide continuing management and therapy.

Genetic Counselor

- Detailed medical/surgical history.
- 3–4 generations pedigree.
- Provide information about recurrence risk.
- Inform about reproductive options (preimplantation diagnosis, prenatal diagnosis, etc.).

How to Find a Medical Geneticist

Information about the location of genetic clinics worldwide can be found on the GeneClinics website at: www.geneclinics.org (this site also has information about where to order genetic tests as well as excellent disease reviews). Clinics in the United States can be found by using the American College of Medical search engine at: www.acmg.net/GIS/. Individual Geneticists in the United States can be located on the websites of the American Board of Medical Genetics and the American College of Medical Genetics:

www.abmg.org
www.acmg.net

Individual Genetic Counselors can be located using the websites of the National Society of Genetic Counselors or the American Board of Genetic Counseling:

www.nsgc.org
www.abgc.net

Reference

1 Pletcher BA, Toriello HV, Noblin SJ, Seaver LH, Driscoll DA, Bennett RL, Gross SJ: Indications for genetic referral: a guide for healthcare providers. Genet Med 2007;9:385–389.

V. Reid Sutton, MD
Texas Children's Hospital
6701 Fannin Suite 1560.10
Houston, TX 77030 (USA)
Tel. +1 832 822 4292, Fax +1 832 825 4294, E-Mail vrsutton@texaschildrens.org

Alford RL, Sutton VR (eds): Medical Genetics in the Clinical Practice of ORL.
Adv Otorhinolaryngol. Basel, Karger, 2011, vol 70, pp 28–36

Towards an Etiologic Diagnosis: Assessing the Patient with Hearing Loss

Jerry Lin[a] · John S. Oghalai[b]

[a]The Bobby R. Alford Department of Otolaryngology, Head and Neck Surgery, Baylor College of Medicine and The Hearing Center at Texas Children's Hospital, Houston, Tex.; [b]Department of Otolaryngology, Head and Neck Surgery, Stanford University and The Children's Hearing Center at Lucile Packard Children's Hospital, Palo Alto, Calif., USA

Abstract

This article reviews the clinical approach taken towards identification of the cause of hearing loss in children. A brief overview of the universal newborn hearing screening program is presented. Discussion is then focused on clinical elements of the diagnostic process with emphasis on the importance of the history, physical examination, and audiologic testing. The utility and appropriateness of additional diagnostic testing is considered, particularly with regards to the incorporation of diagnostic radiologic imaging and genetic testing. In the course of these discussions, the genetic and nongenetic causes of pediatric hearing loss are reviewed. Finally, the implications of a definitive identification of hearing loss etiology are considered.

Hearing loss is the fourth most common developmental disorder in the United States, and deafness is the most common sensory disorder. In the United States, the incidence of congenital hearing loss based on universal neonatal screening programs is estimated to be 1.1 per 1,000 with a range of 0.22–3.61 per 1,000 between individual states [1]. Indigent patients are at a higher risk of neonatal hearing loss than the average US population [2].

Generally, it is estimated that 50% of cases of congenital hearing loss are genetic in nature, 25% are acquired, and the remaining 25% are idiopathic. Of genetic causes for congenital hearing loss, approximately 30% are syndromic, and 70% are nonsyndromic [3]. Genetic causes can also be subdivided by inheritance pattern; approximately 77% of cases are autosomal recessive, 22% are autosomal dominant, 1% are X-linked, and <1% are passed via mitochondrial inheritance from the mother [4].

Prelingual deafness is particularly worrisome as it can engender many other disabilities. The ability to hear during the early years of life is critical for the development of speech, language, and cognition. Hearing impairment is also associated with a reduction in visual reception and fine motor skills as the child ages [5]. Early identification and intervention can prevent severe psychosocial, educational, and linguistic repercussions [6, 7]. The prevalence of congenital hearing loss is greater than twice that of all other diseases and syndromes routinely screened at birth combined [8]. Hence, universal newborn hearing screening programs have been implemented in most states across the country.

Universal Newborn Hearing Screening

As recently as 1988, the Commission on Education of the Deaf estimated that in the United States, congenital hearing loss was diagnosed in children at an average age of 2.5–3 years, a point in time significantly after the onset of the critical period for speech and language development [9]. At that time, the only children screened for hearing loss were those with significant risk factors as defined by the Joint Committee on Infant Hearing (JCIH) [10]. This directed method of screening missed cases of nonsyndromic sensorineural hearing loss (SNHL) and only identified about half of the children who had hearing loss [11]. In 1993, via a consensus statement, the National Institute of Health (NIH) advocated early detection of hearing loss not only in high-risk infants but universally in all infants before 3 months of age [12]. Presently, the JCIH endorses universal screening within a state-run system of early hearing detection and intervention (EHDI). This program has three goals: (1) to identify children with hearing loss by one month of age, (2) to formally diagnose children with hearing loss by three months, and (3) to intervene by 6 months [13].

Initial screening in healthy infants is typically performed using otoacoustic emissions (OAE) testing. A passing OAE result signifies proper functioning of the outer hair cells and the endocochlear potential within the cochlea and is usually interpreted as hearing sensitivity of 30 dB or better. If a child fails an OAE test, an auditory brainstem response (ABR) test is performed. Failing both elements of the hearing screening results in a referral to an audiologist for formal evaluation by 3 months of age.

Typically, ABR abnormalities are associated with a lack of OAE response. In some cases, however, a child will fail an ABR despite passing their OAE testing. This finding suggests auditory neuropathy/dysynchrony, a condition whereby the outer hair cells of the cochlea respond appropriately to auditory input but either the inner hair cells are unable to transduce the signals to the auditory nerve or there is dysfunction of the auditory nerve/brainstem pathways. Since auditory neuropathy/dysynchrony is particularly common in infants within the neonatal intensive care unit (NICU), it is recommended that all infants within the NICU undergo hearing screening using ABR alone [14].

The Colorado hearing screening program has reported that 98% of newborns in the state were screened for hearing loss between 2002–2004 [15]. While the screening rate is high, the remaining percentage of unscreened newborns still represents more than 200,000 children. Therefore, even during regularly scheduled well-child visits, the physician should be vigilant in monitoring the achievement of speech and language developmental milestones in an effort to detect previously missed or progressive hearing loss. The American Speech-Language-Hearing Association summarizes key speech and language developmental milestones on their website [16].

Diagnosing the Etiology of Hearing Loss

Presently, no formal consensus exists regarding which specific diagnostic tests should be ordered for pediatric hearing loss, but all otolaryngologists agree that a careful and complete history and physical examination along with the audiometric data are critical first steps towards diagnosing the cause of a child's hearing loss.

History

The important elements of the history are summarized in table 1. Non-genetic causes of hearing loss can often be revealed during history taking. These acquired causes can be classified into several general categories: (1) infection, (2) prematurity/NICU admission, and (3) miscellaneous.

Infection once comprised the majority of acquired causes of hearing loss. Prenatally, any of the common maternal infections (toxoplasmosis,

Table 1. Elements of history taking for pediatric hearing loss

Prenatal
Maternal infections
Toxoplasmosis, rubella, cytomegalovirus, herpes simplex, syphilis
Maternal medications
Aminoglycosides, quinine, cloroquine, thalidomide
Maternal illnesses
Diabetes
Perinatal
Prematurity
Low birth weight
Birth hypoxia (low APGAR scores)
Hyperbilirubinemia
Sepsis
NICU admission
Ototoxic medications
Postnatal
Viral illnesses (mumps, measles, chicken pox)
Bacterial meningitis
Recurrent or persistent otitis media with effusion
Head trauma
Noise trauma
Neurodegenerative disorders
Speech and language developmental milestones
Family history
First and second-degree relatives with hearing loss
Common origin from ethnically isolated areas
Consanguinity

rubella, cytomegalovirus (CMV), herpes simplex, and syphilis) can manifest as hearing loss. Postnatally, viral illnesses and bacterial meningitis are causes of hearing loss. Advancements in prenatal and neonatal care and the institution of universal immunization programs have decreased the incidence of hearing loss from infectious etiology [17]. In particular, vaccination programs have nearly eliminated congenital rubella and H. influenza type B as significant causes of hearing loss [18, 19]. On the other hand, CMV infection is the most common infectious cause of congenital hearing loss and may be responsible for 12–25% of pediatric hearing loss [20].

As survival rates of premature infants have increased, hearing loss related to prematurity and NICU admissions have become more prevalent. It is not always apparent how prematurity or NICU care directly leads to hearing loss, but children in the NICU typically share one or more of the following traits: birth weight <1,500 g, low APGAR scores (0–3 at 5 min, 0–6 at 10 min), hypoxia requiring respiratory support, hyperbilirubinemia at levels requiring exchange transfusion, sepsis, and exposure to ototoxic medications such as aminoglycoside antibiotics or diuretics [21]. Most often, the hearing loss in these cases is sensorineural and permanent. There is some evidence, however, that correction of hyperbilirubinemia may improve hearing [22].

Other miscellaneous acquired causes of hearing loss that may be suspected after taking a history include chronic otitis media with effusion, congenital stapes fixation, ossicular chain malformation, congenital aural atresia, noise exposure, and head trauma.

Genetic causes of hearing loss are less easily identified by history, but occasionally other elements of a syndromic hearing loss may by identified. These include a history of visual impairment, kidney disease, or syncope spells. Attention to achievement of speech and language developmental milestones may reveal whether the hearing loss was present at birth or later in onset, and whether the hearing loss is progressive in nature.

Non-syndromic genetic hearing loss is far more difficult to identify by history alone. If hearing loss can be adequately identified in first and second degree relatives, constructing a pedigree may identify a pattern of inheritance. Also, children from consanguineous marriages or from family backgrounds arising from small, ethnically homogeneous areas such as Ashkenazi Jews or

Japanese are more likely to suffer from a genetic form of hearing loss [23].

Physical Examination
The physical examination typically performed by an otolaryngologist is in actuality quite limited. Assessments are made of head size and symmetry, jaw size and symmetry, facial movement and symmetry, and external and middle ear morphology. These elements of the physical examination can often reveal pathology associated with acquired causes of hearing loss, particularly those that result in a conductive hearing loss. Examples include middle ear effusion, microtia, external canal atresia, cleft lip or palate, and craniofacial anomalies such as microcephaly, craniosynostosis, micrognathia, or facial asymmetry.

In other cases of congenital hearing loss, associated physical anomalies, particularly in the head and neck region, may be subtle or even nonexistent. Congenital hearing loss can result from one of more than 400 syndromes and be associated with defects in virtually any organ system (reviewed by Toriello et al. [24]). Collaboration between specialists therefore is essential to identify a syndrome.

Audiologic Studies
In neonates, an ABR can give accurate hearing thresholds between 1 and 4 kHz [25]. Auditory steady-state evoked potentials (ASSR) can measure auditory thresholds at levels higher than that often available clinically for ABR [26]. In older children, a behavioral audiogram can be obtained by means of visual reinforcement or conditioned play audiometry. Acquired hearing loss and syndromic genetic hearing loss can be associated with conductive, sensorineural, or mixed forms of hearing loss, but non-syndromic genetic hearing loss is almost always sensorineural. The shape of the audiogram can be used for audiometric profiling, a method that pairs a given frequency response curve with the most likely causative gene mutations [27].

Ancillary Studies
While a history, physical exam, and audiologic evaluation are mandatory in the workup of pediatric hearing loss, the decision to pursue further diagnostic testing is controversial. Some clinicians order an exhaustive array of tests to aid in diagnosis. Others select a few specific tests that may be of higher yield given particular findings on history or physical exam. Despite several studies to determine the usefulness of various sets of diagnostic tests, no consensus exists regarding the appropriate test battery for pediatric hearing loss [28]. Table 2 lists commonly ordered ancillary diagnostic tests.

Imaging Studies
Diagnostic imaging is the most useful ancillary test in determining the cause of pediatric hearing loss. Diagnostic imaging typically consists of computed tomography (CT) of the temporal bone, magnetic resonance imaging (MRI) of the brain and internal auditory canal (IAC), or both. Studies have shown that 27–39% of children with hearing loss who undergo diagnostic imaging will demonstrate an anatomic abnormality that may explain the hearing loss [30, 31]. The most common temporal bone abnormality is an enlarged vestibular aqueduct (EVA). This may or may not be associated with a Mondini malformation in the cochlea and is suggestive of Pendred or Branchio-Oto-Renal syndromes. Other temporal bone anomalies include lateral semicircular canal dysplasia, small IACs, hypoplastic cochleas, and otic capsule lucencies [29]. Figure 1 demonstrates a variety of temporal bone malformations encountered in children with congenital hearing loss.

In many cases, temporal bone anomalies may not be pathognomonic for particular syndromes but may predict clinical course or surgical outcomes. For instance, children with EVA may show progressive sensorineural hearing loss, particularly after mild head trauma [30]. Children with abnormal connections between otic capsule structures and the middle ear may

Table 2. Commonly ordered ancillary studies or consultations in the diagnostic workup for congenital pediatric hearing loss

Study or consultation	Associated etiology for hearing loss
ANA, ESR, RF, anticardiolipin, immunoglobulins, complement studies	autoimmune disease
CBC	thallasemia, Sickle cell anemia
Platelet count	Fechtner syndrome, Epstein syndrome
BUN, creatinine	Alport syndrome*
Glucose	Alstrom syndrome*, diabetes mellitus
Urinalysis	Alport syndrome, metabolic disorders
Antibody titers	toxoplasmosis, rubella, CMV, herpes simplex
FT4, T3, TSH, perchlorate test	Pendred syndrome*, cretinism
RPR, FT-ABS	syphilis
ECG	Jervell Lange-Nielsen syndrome
CT Temporal Bone	temporal bone anomalies
MRI Brain and IAC	cochlear nerve hypoplasia/aplasia, CPA mass, brain lesions
Renal ultrasound	branchio-oto-renal syndrome
Connexin 26/30 genetic testing	connexin 26/30 mutation
Genetics consultation	any genetic etiology
Ophthalmology consultation	Usher syndrome*, Alport syndrome, Cogan's syndrome, Norrie disease, Stickler syndrome

* Note that certain phenotypic features, such as goiter in Pendred syndrome and retinitis pigmentosa in Usher syndrome develop with age and would not be expected to be seen in an infant, thus a normal result would not exclude such a diagnosis in an infant or young child.

be prone to hearing loss, vestibular symptoms, or facial paralysis during occurrences of otitis media. Abnormal connections between the cerebrospinal fluid (CSF) space and inner ear structures such as EVA or absent bone at the modiolus may predispose patients to CSF gushers during and CSF leaks after certain ear surgeries [31]. These patients may also be more prone to meningitis. For patients who have had a history of meningitis, imaging may reveal labyrinthitis ossificans, a condition that complicates placement of a cochlear implant [32].

Renal ultrasound is a commonly performed diagnostic imaging procedure in the workup of pediatric hearing loss [33]. A renal ultrasound is ordered in suspected cases of BOR syndrome looking for developmental renal anomalies.

Laboratory Studies

Many studies suggest that performing a standard battery of laboratory tests is not particularly useful in identifying the etiology for hearing loss. Rather than blanketing all deaf children with multiple blood tests, it has been recommended that specific laboratory tests be ordered on the basis of the patient's history, physical examination, and audiogram [28]. Laboratory tests that are typically ordered to evaluate pediatric hearing loss include complete blood count, serum chemistry panels, thyroid function tests, antibody

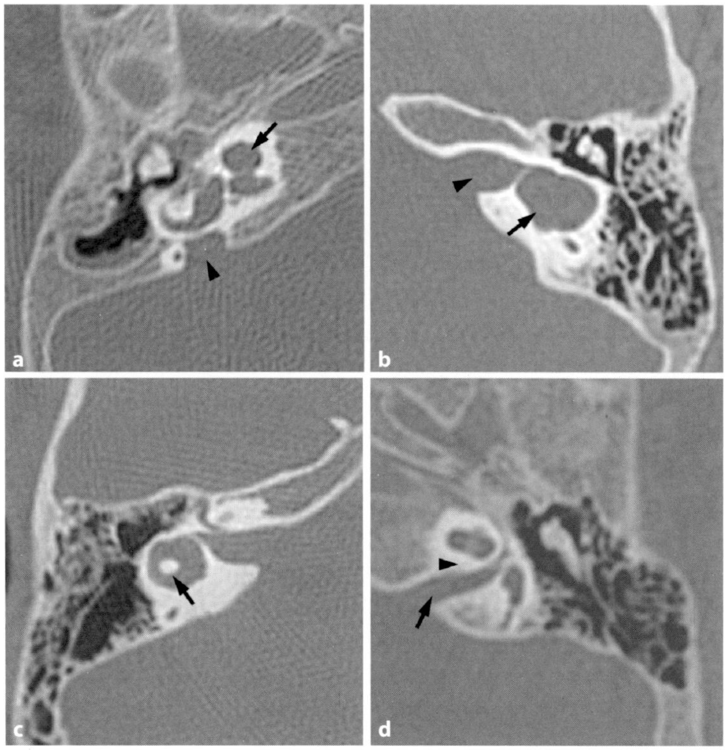

Fig. 1. A variety of CT temporal bone images showing anomalies encountered in children with congenital hearing loss. **a** Axial CT of a right temporal bone with a Mondini malformation of the cochlea (arrow) and an enlarged vestibular aqueduct (arrowhead). **b** Axial CT of a left temporal bone with a common cavity malformation (arrow) and bony separation of common cavity from the IAC (arrowhead). **c** Axial CT of a right temporal bone with lateral semicircular canal dysplasia – the bone island in the center of the canal (arrow) is too small. **d** Axial CT of a left temporal bone with a narrow IAC (arrow) and no cochlear aperture for the auditory nerve to enter the cochlea (expected location is marked by arrowhead).

titers for pre- or perinatal pathogens, autoimmune serologies, and urinalysis. Abnormal laboratory findings for autoimmune serologies occur nearly 25% of the time but are almost never helpful in determining the cause of the hearing loss [28].

Electrocardiography (ECG)
Electrocardiography has a diagnostic yield akin to laboratory testing but deserves mention because of the dire consequences of a missed diagnosis of Jervell and Lange-Nielsen syndrome. This syndrome, which includes deafness and prolonged QT intervals, may initially present as sudden death. An ECG may be obtained in any child with hearing loss to evaluate for this possibility, but would be particularly relevant in a child with a history of syncopal episodes or a family history of sudden infant death syndrome.

Consultations
Hearing loss is disproportionately associated with abnormalities of ocular structures. Therefore, most children with congenital hearing loss are also referred to an ophthalmologist, who can identify subtle ocular abnormalities such as retinitis pigmentosa that may indicate a particular etiology for the hearing loss. Children with nonsyndromic congenital hearing loss can experience decreased visual reception skills as they age [5]. Therefore, at the very least, the child's visual acuity can be evaluated and optimized in order to minimize his or her sensory disabilities and maximize the potential for normal development.

Determining a possible syndromic etiology for hearing loss sometimes requires a familiarity with the constellation of physical findings beyond that of an otolaryngologist. Thus the expertise of a clinical geneticist can be helpful for making a clinical diagnosis of syndromic hearing loss and for pedigree analysis for non-syndromic hearing loss.

Genetic Testing
As our understanding of the molecular basis of hearing improves, a significant percentage of hearing loss that is presently idiopathic will likely be found to have a genetic basis. Non-syndromic hearing loss, which lacks associated physical findings, has typically been a diagnosis of exclusion. In the last 5 years, however, rapid escalation in the numbers of genes found to be responsible for non-syndromic hearing loss has made a definitive diagnosis more likely [34].

The finding in 1997 that up to 50% of autosomal recessive non-syndromic hearing loss in some populations may be due to mutations in the *GJB2* gene that encodes Connexin 26 significantly improved the prospects of genetic testing for hearing loss [35]. Aside from Connexin 26, however, no consensus exists regarding which additional genes should be considered as part of routine testing. In an excellent review of the genetic approach toward diagnosing pediatric hearing loss, Rehm [36] proposes an algorithm that accounts for patterns of inheritance, timing of hearing loss, audiogram profile, and associated clinical findings in recommending specific genes to be tested. This algorithm will evolve as new genes are discovered, functions of existing gene products are revealed, and the prevalences of mutations in known genes are defined. On the other hand, cost reductions and advances in gene testing technology are likely to soon render obsolete any need for algorithmic testing.

Implications of Diagnosis

Every patient or family has different experiences with hearing loss, different attitudes towards genetic testing, and different expectations regarding the outcomes of genetic testing. Therefore, it is imperative to consult a genetic counselor that has experience in dealing with perceptions or misperceptions of genetic testing and managing expectations from testing results. In many instances, finding a genetic basis does not substantially change the patient's treatment or prognosis, at present. Thus, some patients may consider genetic testing to be wasted effort; others, however, may appreciate an identifiable reason for their hearing loss. Parents who are considering having more children might benefit from knowing the inheritance pattern of hearing loss in their family and the likelihood that additional children will be deaf. In other instances, finding a genetic basis for hearing loss may indeed significantly impact a patient's prognosis and management. For example, the diagnosis of Usher syndrome and its associated imminent blindness will direct a patient to concentrate on developing verbal rather than visual means of communication. A finding of mutations in the *12SrRNA* gene allows a patient or patient's family to recognize his or her susceptibility to aminoglycoside-induced hearing loss and to avoid aminoglycoside antibiotics use if possible. In a child with otoferlin mutations, auditory neuropathy/dyssynchrony would be established as the cause of hearing loss and in appropriate circumstances, rehabilitation might be more successful with cochlear implantation rather than hearing aids [37].

Conclusions

Significant advancements have been made in identifying genes important for hearing and understanding of the molecular function of these gene products. For neonatal hearing loss that is acquired or genetic hearing loss that is part of a syndrome, a thoughtful integration of the clinical history, the physical examination, and the audiologic testing may yield a diagnosis of etiology. Genetic testing offers the best chance for determining an etiology for non-syndromic hearing loss. An algorithm integrating our understanding of gene function with clinical findings can be used to select candidate genes that are most likely to be mutated. As more hearing genes are identified and their functions are elucidated, algorithms for genetic testing will become more refined and directed. Concomitantly, improvements in technology will allow for faster more cost-effective genetic testing.

References

1 Mehra S, Eavey RD, Keamy DG: The epidemiology of hearing impairment in the United States: newborns, children, and adolescents. Otolaryngol Head Neck Surg 2009;140:461–472.
2 Oghalai JS, et al: Neonatal hearing loss in the indigent. Laryngoscope 2002;112: 281–286.
3 Hone SW, Smith RJH: Medical evaluation of pediatric hearing loss: laboratory, radiographic, and genetic testing. Otolaryngol Clin N Am 2002;35:751–764.
4 Morton NE: Genetic epidemiology of hearing impairment. Ann NY Acad Sci 1991;630:16–31.
5 Pierson SK, Caudle SE, Krull KR, et al: Cognition in children with sensorineural hearing loss: etiologic considerations. Laryngoscope 2007;117:1661–1665.
6 Robinshaw HM: Early intervention for hearing impairment: differences in the timing of communicative and linguistic development. Br J Audiol 1995;29:315–334.
7 Yoshinaga-Itano C, et al: Language of early- and later-identified children with hearing loss. Pediatrics 1998;102:1161–1171.
8 Finitzo T, Crumley WG: The role of the pediatrician in hearing loss: from detection to connection. Pediatr Clin North Am 1999;46:15–34.
9 Commission on Education of the Deaf: Toward Equality: Education of the Deaf. Washington, 1988.
10 Joint Committee on Infant Hearing: 1990 position statement. Am Speech/Language Hearing Assoc 1991;33(suppl 5):3–6.
11 Mauk GW, White KR, Mortensen LB, et al: The effectiveness of screening programs based on high-risk characteristics in early identification of hearing impairment. Ear Hear 1991;12:312–319.
12 National Institutes of Health: Early Identification of Hearing Impairment in Infants and Young Children: NIH Consensus Development Conference Statement. Bethesda, National Institutes of Health, 1993;pp 1–24.
13 Joint Committee on Infant Hearing: 2007 position statement. Pediatrics 2007;120:898–921.
14 Cristobal R, Oghalai JS: Hearing loss in children with very low birth weight: current review of epidemiology and pathophysiology. Arch Dis Child Fetal Neonatal Ed 2008;93:f462–f468.
15 Christensen M, Thomson V, Letson GW: Evaluating the reach of universal newborn hearing screening in Colorado. Am J Prev Med 2008;359:594–597.
16 http://www.asha.org/public/speech/development/chart.htm.
17 Catlin FI: Prevention of hearing impairment from infection and ototoxic drugs. Arch Otolaryngol 1985;111:377–384.
18 Centers for Disease Control and Prevention: Progress toward elimination of rubella and congenital rubella syndrome – the Americas, 2003–2008. Morb Mortal Wkly Rep 2008;57:1176–1179.
19 Peltola H: Worldwide *Haemophilus influenzae* type B diseases at the beginning of the 21st century: global analysis of the disease burden 25 years after the use of the polysaccharide vaccine and a decade after the advent of conjugates. Clin Microbiol Rev 2000;13:302–317.
20 Fowler KB, Boppana SB: Congenital cytomegalovirus (CMV) infection and hearing deficit. J Clin Virol 2006;35:226–231.
21 Bamiou DE, Macardle B, Bitner-Glindzicz M, et al: Aetiological investigations of hearing loss in childhood: a review. Clin Otolaryngol 2000;25:98–106.
22 Kuriyama M, Tomiwa K, Konishi Y, et al: Improvement in auditory brainstem response of hyperbilirubinemic infants after exchange transfusions. Pediatr Neurol 1986;2:127–132.
23 Basil A: Childhood sensorineural hearing loss in consanguineous marriages. J Audiol Med 1994;3:151–159.
24 Toriello HV, Reardon W, Gorlin RJ: Hereditary Hearing Loss and Its Syndromes, ed 2. Oxford, Oxford University Press, 1995.
25 Tomaski SM, Grundfast KM: A stepwise approach to the diagnosis and treatment of hereditary hearing loss. Pediatr Clin N Am 1999;46:35–47.
26 Oghalai JS, Tonini R, Rasmus J, et al: Intra-operative monitoring of cochlear function during cochlear implantation. Cochlear Implants Int 2009;10:1–18.
27 Hildebrand MS, DeLuca AP, Taylor KR, et al: A contemporary review of Audiogene audioprofiling: a machine-based candidate gene prediction tool for autosomal dominant nonsyndromic hearing loss. Laryngoscope 2009;119: 2211–2215.
28 Mafong DD, Shin EJ, Lalwani AK: Use of laboratory evaluation and radiologic imaging in the diagnostic evaluation of children with sensorineural hearing loss. Laryngoscope 2002;112:1–7.
29 Antonelli PJ, Varela AE, Mancuso AA: Diagnostic yield of high-resolution computed tomography for pediatric sensorineural hearing loss. Laryngoscope 1999;109:1642–1647.
30 Madden C, Halsted M, Benton C, et al: Enlarged vestibular aqueduct syndrome in the pediatric population. Oto Neurotol 2003;24:625–632.
31 Luntz M, Balkany T, Hodges AV, et al: Cochlear implants in children with congenital inner ear malformation. Arch Otolaryngol Head Neck Surg 1997;123: 974–977.

32 Philipon D, Bergeron F, Ferron P, et al: Cochlear implantation in postmeningitic deafness. Oto Neurotol 2010;31:83–87.
33 Wang RY, Dawn LE, Ruder RO, et al: Sydromic ear anomalies and renal ultrasounds. Pediatrics 2001;108:E32.
34 Hilgert N, Smith RJH, Van Camp G: Function and expression pattern of non-syndromic deafness genes. Curr Mol Med 2009;9:546–564.
35 Kelsell DP, Dunlop J, Stevens HP, et al: Connexin 26 mutationsin hereditary non-syndromic sensorineural deafness. Nature 1997;387:80–83.
36 Rehm HL: A genetic approach to the child with sensorineural hearing loss. Semin Perinatol 2005;29:173–181.
37 Berlin CI, Hood LJ, Morlet T, et al: Multi-site diagnosis and management of 260 patients with auditory neuropathy/dys-synchrony (auditory neuropathy spectrum disorder). Int J Audiol 2010; 49:30–43.

John S. Oghalai, MD
Department of Otolaryngology, Head and Neck Surgery, Stanford University
801 Welch Road
Stanford, CA 94305–5739 (USA)
Tel. +1 650 725 6500, Fax +1 650 721 2163, E-Mail joghalai@ohns.stanford.edu

Alford RL, Sutton VR (eds): Medical Genetics in the Clinical Practice of ORL.
Adv Otorhinolaryngol. Basel, Karger, 2011, vol 70, pp 37–42

Nonsyndromic Hereditary Hearing Loss

Raye L. Alford

Bobby R. Alford Department of Otolaryngology – Head and Neck Surgery, Baylor College of Medicine, Houston, Tex., USA

Abstract

The etiology of hereditary hearing loss is extraordinarily complex. More than 400 genetic syndromes are associated with hearing loss and more than 140 genetic loci associated with nonsyndromic hearing loss have been mapped, with more than 60 genes identified to date. Hereditary hearing loss can be inherited as an autosomal dominant, autosomal recessive, X-linked or mitochondrial (maternally inherited) condition. The overlapping audiologic phenotypes associated with many genes and the variability and/or reduced, sometimes age-related, penetrance of some phenotypic features of syndromic hearing loss can complicate the distinction between various genetic causes of nonsyndromic hearing loss and between nonsyndromic and syndromic hearing loss, especially in childhood. Testing for individual genes associated with nonsyndromic hearing loss, beyond *GJB2* which encodes Connexin 26, can become expensive and, without specific phenotypic features to guide selection of genes for testing (such as enlarged vestibular aqueducts, low frequency hearing loss or auditory neuropathy), it is not likely to yield an etiology. Advances in DNA sequencing and the rapid decline in the cost of sequencing presage the availability of testing that can identify the etiology in the majority of cases of genetic hearing loss. However, until comprehensive genetic testing of hearing loss is clinically available and cost-effective, thorough phenotypic and audiologic evaluation and careful documentation of risk factors, infectious exposures and patient and family medical history will continue to be important to efforts directed toward etiologic diagnosis. The complexities associated with interpretation of genetic test results, genetic counseling and genetic risk assessment make consultation with medical geneticists important for many patients.

So you have been asked to evaluate a patient with hearing loss. After a variety of assessments, you rule out common risk factors and infectious etiologies, document an absence of features associated with syndromic hearing loss, and elicit a negative family history. Now what?

This scenario is not uncommon. The prospect of identifying an etiologic cause for a presumptive nonsyndromic hereditary hearing loss (NSHHL) can be daunting. The number of genes involved, overlapping auditory phenotypes associated with many genes, variability and/or reduced, sometimes age-related, penetrance of some features of syndromic hearing loss, and lack of availability and/or expense of some genetic tests preclude an etiologic diagnosis for many patients. However, etiologic diagnosis is important and can provide prognostic information about the hearing loss and whether a patient is at increased risk for other medical problems associated with syndromic hearing loss. Etiologic diagnosis also offers patients an explanation for the hearing loss, informs genetic counseling and genetic risk assessment for patients and relatives, and aids in the establishment of a treatment and management plan [1].

As discussed in the chapter by Lin and Oghalai [this vol.], a number of clinical assessments can aid in the etiologic diagnosis of hearing loss. In 2002, the American College of Medical Genetics (ACMG) issued 'Genetics evaluation guidelines for the etiologic diagnosis of congenital hearing loss' which outlined various clinical assessments relevant to hearing impaired patients including medical genetic evaluation and genetic testing [1]. These guidelines can arguably be extrapolated, with some modifications, to patients with later onset hearing loss.

Genetic testing is a powerful tool for the etiologic diagnosis of hearing loss [1, 2]. A number of questions can aid in the selection of genes for testing such as: is there a relevant family history; are there developmental, morphological or other abnormalities or signs of a syndrome; and, what is the audiologic profile, that is, what is the age of onset, symmetry and degree of hearing loss, is the loss sensorineural, conductive, mixed, progressive, what frequencies of sound are affected, is there auditory neuropathy?

Autosomal Dominant NSHHL

Autosomal dominant NSHHL typically presents with a family history consistent with autosomal dominant inheritance [see chapter by Alford and Darilek, this vol.], however, because *de novo* mutations can occur, some patients may not have a positive family history. Further, assortative mating among deaf individuals could result in both parents being hearing impaired due to any number of causes, thus complicating the use of pedigree analysis in determining the pattern of inheritance. Presently, 61 loci associated with autosomal dominant NSHHL have been mapped with 24 causative genes identified [3]. In general, autosomal dominant NSHHL tends to affect predominantly higher frequencies of sound, be progressive and sensorineural, have a wide range of age of onset, and trend toward post-lingual onset, although pre-lingual onset has been reported with a few genes including *GJB2, TECTA*, and possibly *COL11A2* [2, 4–7].

Vestibular dysfunction and/or tinnitus have been reported in association with several genes including *COCH* and *WFS1* [8, 9]. In addition, some genes are associated with unusual audiometric phenotypes which are particularly evident in early stages of the hearing loss and offer the opportunity for targeted genetic testing. For example, *DIAPH1* and *WFS1* are associated with low-frequency hearing loss, *COL11A2, TECTA* and *EYA4* are associated with mid-frequency hearing loss, *CCDC50* is associated with low- to mid-frequency hearing loss, and *DIAPH3* is associated with autosomal dominant auditory neuropathy [2, 4, 9–17].

Autosomal Recessive NSHHL

Autosomal recessive NSHHL typically presents with a family history consistent with an autosomal recessive pattern of inheritance [see chapter by Alford and Darilek, this vol.], however, the commonness of some etiologies and assortative mating among deaf individuals could result in one or both parents being hearing impaired. In such cases, one might assume that if a child and one or both parents are affected with NSHHL, the condition is being transmitted in a dominant manner; however, given the high frequency of recessive *GJB2*-related NSHHL, this is not necessarily the case. This phenomenon, known as pseudodominant inheritance, was discussed in detail in the chapter by Alford and Darilek [this vol.]. Presently, 81 loci associated with autosomal recessive NSHHL have been mapped with 36 causative genes identified [3]. In general, autosomal recessive NSHHL tends to be pre-lingual, severe to profound, sensorineural and nonprogressive although postlingual, mild-to-moderate and progressive hearing loss have been reported [2].

In particular, the DFNB1 locus warrants special mention. Mutations in two genes residing at this locus, *GJB2*, which encodes the protein connexin 26, and *GJB6*, which encodes the protein connexin 30, may cause up to 50% of autosomal recessive NSHHL in some populations. Carrier rates for recessive mutations in *GJB2* range from 4.76% in Ashkenazi Jews to 3% in Caucasians and 1% in Asians [18–23]. Autosomal recessive NSHHL associated with the DFNB1 locus can be caused by biallelic mutations in *GJB2*, biallelic deletions in *GJB6*, or heterozygous mutation in *GJB2* and deletion in *GJB6* [23–26]. Although NSHHL caused by mutations in *GJB2* and *GJB6* is typically recessive, congenital, nonprogressive and severe-to-profound, rare dominant mutations in *GJB2* and *GJB6* have been reported, and mild-to-moderate and possibly progressive NSHHL and syndromic hearing loss have been reported with mutations in *GJB2* [23].

Two findings that may be associated with autosomal recessive NSHHL offer the opportunity for targeted genetic testing. These include enlarged vestibular aqueduct which is associated with mutations in *SLC26A4* and auditory neuropathy which is associated with mutations in *OTOF* and *PJVK* [27–30]. Individually, other autosomal recessive NSHHL genes account for only a small fraction of cases. As such, the cost-benefit ratio of genetic testing beyond *GJB2* and *GJB6* in cases lacking enlarged vestibular aqueducts or auditory neuropathy is presently unfavorable although this is likely to change in the next few years as affordable multiplex testing becomes available.

X-Linked NSHHL

X-linked NSHHL typically presents with a family history consistent with an X-linked pattern of inheritance [see chapter by Alford and Darilek, this vol.]; however, small family size, which limits the potential for an affected male relative, and *de novo* mutations might result in a negative family history. Presently, 5 loci associated with X-linked NSHHL have been mapped and 2 causative genes identified [3].

Four phenotypes, three of which are syndromic, are associated with mutations in *PRPS1* [31]. NSHHL associated with mutations in *PRPS1* ranges in age of onset from the first to second decade for males, may be progressive, and is typically of later onset, milder and may be asymmetric in females [32]. Mutations in *POU3F4* are associated with progressive sensorineural hearing loss, with or without conductive hearing loss due to stapes fixation, and dilatation of the internal acoustic canal with an abnormally wide communication between the internal acoustic canal and the inner ear compartment which predisposes to perilymphatic gusher [33].

Mitochondrial (Maternally Inherited) NSHHL

Mitochondrial NSHHL typically presents with a family history consistent with inheritance along the maternal lineage [see chapter by Alford and Darilek, this vol.]; however, maternally inherited NSHHL can show considerable variability, is often progressive, and may demonstrate reduced penetrance so patients may not report a family history of hearing loss [34, 35]. Presently, 2 mitochondrial genes have been associated with NSHHL [3].

Of particular note, the m.1555A>G mutation in *MTRNR1* is associated with susceptibility to aminoglycoside ototoxicity and with NSHHL without a history of exposure to aminoglycosides [34, 35]. Mutations in *MTTS1* are associated with NSHHL and syndromic hearing loss [34, 36]. Besides the m.1555A>G mutation in *MTRNR1*, other mutations in both *MTRNR1* and *MTTS1* have been reported in association with aminoglycoside ototoxicity; however, the clinical significance of these variants is not entirely clear [34, 36, 37]. For mutations associated with aminoglycoside ototoxicity, the age of onset of hearing loss is often reduced and progression is accelerated by exposure [34, 35].

Importance of Genetics Consultation

Thorough assessment of patients for syndromic hearing loss may require a more comprehensive examination than can be performed in the otolaryngologist's office. Genetic counseling and genetic risk assessment can be complex. The interpretation of even simple genetic tests is not always straightforward and can change over time. Moreover, genetic testing technologies are changing rapidly, permitting ever more comprehensive testing and ever greater opportunities for etiologic diagnosis; however, these advances also make genetic testing and interpretation of genetic test results more complicated. To interpret genetic test results, physicians need to know whether tests utilize sequencing or allele specific methods, which genes/mutations are included in test panels, which genetic variants are benign polymorphisms and which are pathologic mutations, and how the frequency of alleles in different populations affects interpretation, especially of negative test results. Medical geneticists are an expert resource on matters related to genetic conditions and genetic testing. Consultation with medical geneticists, and other specialists, can be an important part of the evaluation of hearing impaired patients [1]. Clinical geneticists, genetic counselors, genetics clinics, and genetics laboratories can be found through the ACMG, www.acmg.net, GeneTests/GeneClinics, www.genetests.org, and the National Society of Genetic Counselors (NSGC), www.nsgc.org.

Conclusions

Hereditary hearing loss is extremely complex. Advanced genetic testing technologies will soon make comprehensive genetic testing for hearing impaired patients possible and affordable. Evaluation of patients for syndromic hearing loss, selection of appropriate genetic tests, interpretation of genetic test results, genetic counseling, and genetic risk assessment can be complex and may require a multidisciplinary approach. The involvement of medical geneticists in the care of hearing impaired patients and their families offers significant value for patients and physicians.

Note

The rapid pace of discovery in the area of NSHHL demands dynamic resources. The Hereditary Hearing Loss homepage, http://hereditaryhearingloss.org/, Online Mendelian Inheritance in Man (OMIM) database, www.ncbi.nlm.nih.gov/omim, GeneReviews website, www.genetests.org, and Genetics Home Reference, www.ghr.nlm.nih.gov, provide frequently updated information. In addition, many genes and mutations associated with hearing loss have, to date, been detected in only one or a few families. Consequently, little is currently known about the potential range of phenotypes associated with many genes and mutations. Existing knowledge should be expected to evolve as additional patients and families are studied.

References

1 Genetic Evaluation of Congenital Hearing Loss Expert Panel: Genetics evaluation guidelines for the etiologic diagnosis of congenital hearing loss. Genet Med 2004;4:162–171.

2 Smith RJH, Hildebrand MS, Van Camp G: Deafness and hereditary hearing loss overview; in: GeneReviews at GeneTests: Medical Genetics Information Resource (database online). Copyright, University of Washington, Seattle, 1997–2010. Available at http://www.genetests.org.

3 Van Camp G, Smith RJH. Hereditary hearing loss homepage. http://hereditaryhearingloss.org.

4 De Leenheer EM, Kunst HH, McGuirt WT, Prasad SD, Brown MR, Huygen PL, Smith RJ, Cremers CW: Autosomal dominant inherited hearing impairment caused by a missense mutation in COL11A2 (DFNA13). Arch Otolaryngol Head Neck Surg 2001;127:13–17.
5 Denoyelle F, Lina-Granade G, Plauchu H, Bruzzone R, Chaib H, Levi-Acobas F, Weil D, Petit C: Connexin 26 gene linked to a dominant deafness. Nature 1998;393:319–320.
6 Tekin M, Arnos KS, Xia XJ, Oelrich MK, Liu XZ, Nance WE, Pandya A: W44C mutation in the connexin 26 gene associated with dominant non-syndromic deafness. Clin Genet 2001;59:269–273.
7 Verhoeven K, Van Laer L, Kirschhofer K, et al: Mutations in the human alpha-tectorin gene cause autosomal dominant non-syndromic hearing impairment. Nat Genet 1998;19:60–62.
8 Robertson NG, Lu L, Heller S, et al: Mutations in a novel cochlear gene cause DFNA9, a human nonsyndromic deafness with vestibular dysfunction. Nat Genet 1998;20:299–303.
9 Bespalova IN, Van Camp G, Bom SJ, Brown DJ, Cryns K, DeWan AT, Erson AE, Flothmann K, Kunst HP, Kurnool P, Sivakumaran TA, Cremers CW, Leal SM, Burmeister M, Lesperance MM: Mutations in the Wolfram syndrome 1 gene (WFS1) are a common cause of low frequency sensorineural hearing loss. Hum Mol Genet 2001;10:2501–2508.
10 Leon PE, Lalwani AK: Auditory phenotype of DFNA1. Adv Otorhinolaryngol 2002;61:34–40.
11 Lynch ED, Lee MK, Morrow JE, Welcsh PL, Leon PE, King MC: Nonsyndromic deafness DFNA1 associated with mutation of a human homolog of the Drosophila gene diaphanous. Science 1997;278:1315–1318.
12 Modamio-Hoybjor S, Mencia A, Goodyear R, del Castillo I, Richardson G, Moreno F, Moreno-Pelayo MA: A mutation in CCDC50, a gene encoding an effector of epidermal growth factor-mediated cell signaling, causes progressive hearing loss. Am J Hum Genet 2007; 80:1076–1089.
13 Moreno-Pelayo MA, del Castillo I, Villamar M, Romero L, Hernandez-Calvin FJ, Herraiz C, Barbera R, Navas C, Moreno F: A cysteine substitution in the zona pellucida domain of alpha-tectorin results in autosomal dominant, postlingual, progressive, mid frequency hearing loss in a Spanish family. J Med Genet 2001;38:e13.
14 Schoen CJ, Emery SB, Thorne MC, Ammana HR, Sliwerska E, Arnett J, Hortsch M, Hannan F, Burmeister M, Lesperance MM: Increased activity of diaphanous homolog 3 (DIAPH3)/diaphanous causes hearing defects in humans with auditory neuropathy and in *Drosophila*. Proc Natl Acad Sci USA 2010;107:13396–13401.
15 Verhoeven K, Fagerheim T, Prasad S, Wayne S, De Clau F, Balemans W, Verstreken M, Schatteman I, Solem B, Van de Heyning P, Tranebjarg L, Smith RJ, Van Camp G: Refined localization and two additional linked families for the DFNA10 locus for nonsyndromic hearing impairment. Hum Genet 2000; 107:7–11.
16 Wayne S, Robertson NG, DeClau F, Chen N, Verhoeven K, Prasad S, Tranebjarg L, Morton CC, Ryan AF, Van Camp G, Smith RJ: Mutations in the transcriptional activator EYA4 cause late-onset deafness at the DFNA10 locus. Hum Mol Genet 2001;10:195–200.
17 Young TL, Ives E, Lynch E, Person R, Snook S, MacLaren L, Cater T, Griffin A, Fernandez B, Lee MK, King MC: Non-syndromic progressive hearing loss DFNA38 is caused by heterozygous missense mutation in the Wolfram syndrome gene WFS1. Hum Mol Genet 2001;10:2509–2514.
18 Green GE, Scott DA, McDonald JM, Woodworth GG, Sheffield VC, Smith RJ: Carrier rates in the midwestern United States for GJB2 mutations causing inherited deafness. JAMA 1999;281:2211–2216.
19 Liu XZ, Xia XJ, Ke XM, Ouyang XM, Du LL, Liu YH, Angeli S, Telischi FF, Nance WE, Balkany T, Xu LR: The prevalence of connexin 26 (GJB2) mutations in the Chinese population. Hum Genet 2002; 111:394–397.
20 Morell RJ, Kim HJ, Hood LJ, Goforth L, Friderici K, Fisher R, Van Camp G, Berlin CI, Oddoux C, Ostrer H, Keats B, Friedman TB: Mutations in the connexin 26 gene (GJB2) among Ashkenazi Jews with nonsyndromic recessive deafness. N Engl J Med 1998;339:1500–1505.
21 Kudo T, Ikeda K, Kure S, Matsubara Y, Oshima T, Watanabe K, Kawase T, Narisawa K, Takasaka T: Novel mutations in the connexin 26 gene (GJB2) responsible for childhood deafness in the Japanese population. Am J Med Genet 2000;90:141–145.
22 Park HJ, Hahn SH, Chun YM, Park K, Kim HN: Connexin 26 mutations associated with nonsyndromic hearing loss. Laryngoscope 2000;110:1535–1538.
23 Smith RJH, Van Camp G: Nonsyndromic hearing loss and deafness, DFNB1; in: GeneReviews at GeneTests: Medical Genetics Information Resource (database online). Copyright, University of Washington, Seattle, 1997–2010. Available at http://www.genetests.org.
24 Del Castillo FJ, Rodriguez-Ballesteros M, Alvarez A, et al: A novel deletion involving the connexin-30 gene, del(GJB6-d13s1854), found in trans with mutations in the GJB2 gene (connexin-26) in subjects with DFNB1 non-syndromic hearing impairment. J Med Genet 2005; 42:588–594.
25 Lerer I, Sagi M, Ben-Neriah Z, Wang T, Levi H, Abeliovich D: A deletion mutation in GJB6 cooperating with a GJB2 mutation in trans in non-syndromic deafness: a novel founder mutation in Ashkenazi Jews. Hum Mutat 2001; 18:460.
26 Pallares-Ruiz N, Blanchet P, Mondain M, Claustres M, Roux AF: A large deletion including most of GJB6 in recessive non-syndromic deafness: a digenic effect? Eur J Hum Genet 2002;10:72–76.
27 Li XC, Everett LA, Lalwani AK, Desmukh D, Friedman TB, Green ED, Wilcox ER: A mutation in PDS causes non-syndromic recessive deafness. Nat Genet 1998;18:215–217.
28 Pryor SP, Madeo AC, Reynolds JC, Sarlis NJ, Arnos KS, Nance WE, Yang Y, Zalewski CK, Brewer CC, Butman JA, Griffith AJ: SLC26A4/PDS genotype-phenotype correlation in hearing loss with enlargement of the vestibular aqueduct (EVA): evidence that Pendred syndrome and non-syndromic EVA are distinct clinical and genetic entities. J Med Genet 2005;42:159–165.

29 Delmaghani S, Del Castillo FJ, Michel V, Leibovici M, Aghaie A, Ron U, Van Laer L, Ben-Tal N, Van Camp G, Weil D, Langa F, Lathrop M, Avan P, Petit C: Mutations in the gene encoding pejvakin, a newly identified protein of the afferent auditory pathway, cause DFNB59 auditory neuropathy. Nat Genet 2006;38:770–778.
30 Varga R, Kelley PM, Keats BJ, Starr A, Leal SM, Cohn E, Kimberling WJ: Non-syndromic recessive auditory neuropathy is the result of mutations in the otoferlin (OTOF) gene. J Med Genet 2003;40:45–50.
31 Online Mendelian Inheritance in Man, OMIM (TM): Baltimore, Johns Hopkins University, MIM ID: 311850:Phosphoribosylpyrophosphate synthetase 1; PRPS1. http://www.ncbi.nlm.nih.gov/omim.
32 Liu X, Han D, Li J, et al: Loss-of-function mutations in the PRPS1 gene cause a type of nonsyndromic X-linked sensorineural deafness, DFN2. Am J Hum Genet 2010;86:65–71.
33 de Kok YJ, van der Maarel SM, Bitner-Glindzicz M, Huber I, Monaco AP, Malcolm S, Pembrey ME, Ropers HH, Cremers FP: Association between X-linked mixed deafness and mutations in the POU domain gene POU3F4. Science 1995;267:685–688.
34 Pandya A: Nonsyndromic hearing loss and deafness, mitochondrial; in: GeneReviews at GeneTests: Medical Genetics Information Resource (database online). Copyright, University of Washington, Seattle, 1997–2010. Available at http://www.genetests.org.
35 Estivill X, Govea N, Barcelo E, Badenas C, Romero E, Moral L, Scozzri R, D'Urbano L, Zeviani M, Torroni A: Familial progressive sensorineural deafness is mainly due to the mtDNA A1555G mutation and is enhanced by treatment of aminoglycosides. Am J Hum Genet 1998;62:27–35.
36 Online Mendelian Inheritance in Man, OMIM (TM): Baltimore, Johns Hopkins University, MD. MIM ID: 590080:Transfer RNA, Mitochondrial, Serine, 1; MTTS1. http://www.ncbi.nlm.nih.gov/omim.
37 Yao YG, Salas A, Bravi CM, Bandelt HJ: A reappraisal of complete mtDNA variation in East Asian families with hearing impairment. Hum Genet 2006;119:505–515.

Raye L. Alford, PhD, FACMG
Bobby R. Alford Department of Otolaryngology – Head and Neck Surgery
Baylor College of Medicine, One Baylor Plaza, NA102
Houston, TX 77030 (USA)
Tel. +1 713 798 8599, Fax +1 713 798 3403, E-Mail ralford@bcm.edu

Alford RL, Sutton VR (eds): Medical Genetics in the Clinical Practice of ORL.
Adv Otorhinolaryngol. Basel, Karger, 2011, vol 70, pp 43–49

Hereditary Hearing Loss with Thyroid Abnormalities

Byung Yoon Choi[a] · Julie Muskett[b] · Kelly A. King[b] · Christopher K. Zalewski[b] · Thomas Shawker[c] · James C. Reynolds[d] · John A. Butman[c] · Carmen C. Brewer[b] · Andrew K. Stewart[e] · Seth L. Alper[e] · Andrew J. Griffith[b]

[a]Laboratory of Molecular Genetics and [b]Otolaryngology Branch, National Institute on Deafness and Other Communication Disorders, National Institutes of Health, Rockville, Md., [c]Diagnostic Radiology Department and [d]Nuclear Medicine Department, Clinical Center, National Institutes of Health, Bethesda, Md., and [e]Beth Israel Deaconess Medical Center, Harvard Medical School, Boston, Mass., USA

Abstract

Mutations in *SLC26A4* can cause deafness and goiter in Pendred syndrome (PDS) or isolated non-syndromic enlargement of the vestibular aqueduct (NSEVA). PDS is one of the most common hereditary causes of deafness. It is characterized by autosomal-recessive inheritance of sensorineural hearing loss, enlarged vestibular aqueducts (EVA), and an iodide organification defect with or without goiter. The diagnosis is confirmed by detection of two mutant alleles of *SLC26A4* in a patient with EVA. The perchlorate discharge test can detect the underlying thyroid biochemical defect and is useful for the evaluation of goiter or for the clinical diagnosis of PDS in a patient with a non-diagnostic *SLC26A4* genotype. *SLC26A4* encodes the pendrin polypeptide, an anion exchanger that, in recombinant expression systems, transports chloride, bicarbonate, and iodide. Investigation of pendrin function in the inner ear has been facilitated by the *Slc26a4*$^{\Delta}$ (knockout) mouse model, but the exact mechanism of its hearing loss remains unclear, as does pendrin's principal transport function in the inner ear. Treatment of PDS is focused upon rehabilitation of hearing loss, and surveillance and management of goiter and, less commonly, hypothyroidism.

The requirement of thyroxine for development of the inner ear is well established. Hearing loss has been documented in diverse disease entities associated with congenital thyroid dysfunction, such as endemic cretinism, non-endemic congenital hypothyroidism, resistance to thyroid hormone (RTH; OMIM 188570), and Pendred syndrome (PDS; OMIM 274600). The latter two disorders are inherited as Mendelian traits and are the focus of this review. Although mutations in other genes can cause congenital hypothyroidism, the combination of deafness and goiter is typically associated with RTH or PDS.

Resistance to Thyroid Hormone

RTH is a rare autosomal-dominant disease caused by mutations in thyroid hormone receptor-β (*THRB*; OMIM 190160). The phenotype reflects resistance to thyroid hormone in target tissues (RTH; OMIM 188570) [1]. Approximately 20%

of RTH patients have hearing loss which is typically mild [1] and has not been reported in association with radiologically detectable inner ear malformations such as enlargement of the vestibular aqueduct (EVA). The hallmark clinical presentation of RTH is goiter and tachycardia associated with elevated serum thyroid hormone levels and unsuppressed TSH [1]. This distinctive endocrinologic phenotype in combination with a *THRB* mutation and a radiologically normal inner ear distinguishes RTH from PDS and other deafness-goiter disorders.

Pendred Syndrome

In 1896, Vaughan Pendred [2] first described the syndrome of congenital deafness and goiter that now bears his name. The definition of PDS was further refined by introduction of a perchlorate discharge test which revealed a defect in iodide organification in this syndrome [3] and by recognition of enlarged vestibular aqueduct as an important phenotypic feature [4]. Autosomal-recessive inheritance was proposed by Fraser [5] based upon his review of the literature and a comprehensive survey of 207 families. The causative gene was identified as *PDS* (now known as *SLC26A4*) through positional cloning [6]. *SLC26A4* is composed of 21 exons and predicted to encode a 780-amino acid (86-kDa) transmembrane protein designated as pendrin.

Subsequent studies demonstrated that mutations in *SLC26A4* may also be associated with non-syndromic deafness and enlarged vestibular aqueducts not accompanied by goiter and the iodide organification defect (NSEVA) (DFNB4; OMIM 600791) [7, 8]. Whereas PDS is strongly correlated with two mutant alleles of *SLC26A4*, NSEVA can be associated with zero, one or two mutant alleles of *SLC26A4* [9, 10]. Some, if not most, NSEVA cases with no detectable mutation of *SLC26A4* appear to be unlinked to DFNB4 (*SLC26A4*) [9, 11, 12].

Genotypic and phenotypic studies of diverse populations have estimated that 4.7 to 7.8% of hereditary deafness is due to PDS, establishing it as the most common form of syndromic deafness [5, 13–15].

Phenotype: Hearing Loss
The hearing loss in PDS is usually pre- or perilingual in onset, although it is not always congenital. Pure tone audiometry generally reveals downsloping or flat, severe-to-profound, bilateral sensorineural hearing loss, although milder hearing loss has also been reported. The hearing loss can be asymmetric. Progression and fluctuation are common, and progression is most rapid in early childhood [16]. These audiological characteristics are similar to those of NSEVA, in which unilateral hearing impairment can also occur [17].

The frequently observed low-frequency air-bone gaps, in combination with normal tympanometry in PDS/NSEVA patients [18–22] are thought to reflect the presence of a '3rd window' in the inner ear [21]. This is consistent with lower thresholds for the vestibular-evoked myogenic potential in some PDS/NSEVA patients [23].

Phenotype: Radiologic
Enlargement of the vestibular aqueduct (EVA) was first defined as a >1.5 mm diameter of the mid-portion of the descending limb of the vestibular aqueduct [17]. Enlargement of the endolymphatic sac and duct in association with EVA is a completely penetrant feature of PDS when evaluated by both temporal bone CT and magnetic resonance imaging (MRI) [4]. Incomplete partition of the apical turn of cochlea, a hypoplastic modiolus, and vestibular malformations may also be present [24]. EVA associated with more severe inner ear anomalies such as cochlear hypoplasia, superior semicircular canal agenesis, or a common cavity deformity is likely to have an etiology other than *SLC26A4* mutations [25]. There appears to be no correlation of size of the vestibular aqueduct

or of the presence of an incomplete cochlear partition with the degree of hearing loss [22, 26].

Phenotype: Thyroid

Goiter is an incompletely penetrant manifestation of PDS. Indeed, it is absent in many cases [27, 28]. Goiter, if present, usually begins during adolescence [5, 29], making the distinction between PDS and NSEVA difficult during childhood. Most patients are euthyroid, irrespective of the presence of goiter, although subclinical hypothyroidism and TSH levels at the upper range of normal may occur [27, 28, 30].

The perchlorate discharge test has emerged as the most sensitive and specific method to identify the underlying thyroid biochemical defect in PDS [28, 29]. An abnormally high (>15%) discharge of perchlorate is very strongly correlated with two mutant alleles of *SLC26A4*. This test is an important tool for the evaluation of goiter and genetic diagnosis in EVA patients with non-diagnostic *SLC26A4* genotypes [9, 28, 31].

Molecular and Cellular Pathogenesis

Pendrin is a transmembrane protein originally hypothesized to be a sulfate transporter [6], but subsequent studies demonstrated that it transports I^-, Cl^-, HCO_3^- or formate [32–34]. Pendrin is thought to mediate efflux of iodide across the apical surface of thyroid follicular cells [35]. In the mouse inner ear, pendrin is expressed in nonsensory epithelia of the endolymphatic duct and sac, cochlear outer sulcus, and transitional cells of the utricle and saccule [36]. It is thought to play a role in endolymphatic homeostasis since these regions are putatively important for the regulation of endolymphatic fluid composition.

Homozygous *Slc26a4*$^{\Delta}$ (knockout) mice show early-onset profound deafness without a detectable thyroid abnormality [37]. *Slc26a4*$^{\Delta}$ mice have significant endolymphatic hydrops and dilatation of all inner ear structures, a phenotype similar to the enlarged endolymphatic sac and duct of human patients with PDS. Endolymph acidification, free radical oxidative damage, local tissue hypothyroidism and macrophage invasion have all been observed in postnatal *Slc26a4*$^{\Delta}$ cochleae [38–41], but a causal relationship to hearing loss is not clear, and the pathogenesis of hearing loss in PDS remains uncertain.

SLC26A4 *Mutation Testing*

Approximately 200 mutations in the *SLC26A4* gene have been reported in PDS or NSEVA patients (www.healthcare.uiowa.edu/labs/pendredandbor) [42]. Mutations have been identified in every coding exon and splice site. There are significant differences in *SLC26A4* mutant alleles among diverse ethnic groups (see figure 4 in Choi et al. [25]). In comparison to European and other mixed populations characterized by relatively broad mutation distributions, East Asians and Pakistanis have restricted distributions of *SLC26A4* mutations with one or a few highly prevalent founder alleles in each population [13, 15, 25, 43–45]. c.919–2A>G, p.H723R and p.V239D are prevalent founder mutations among Chinese, Japanese/Korean, and Pakistani populations, respectively [13, 25, 43–45]. Hierarchical strategies to preferentially screen or sequence selected exons or specific mutations have been proposed for these populations [13, 15, 25, 46]. In contrast, screening or direct sequencing of all coding exons of *SLC26A4* is recommended for populations with broad mutation distributions.

Genotype-Phenotype Correlation

SLC26A4 mutations are detected both in PDS and NSEVA patients, leading some to conclude that PDS and NSEVA are variable manifestations of the same disease entity [43, 47]. Scott et al. [48] proposed that normal thyroid function in NSEVA patients is the consequence of residual pendrin activity encoded by hypofunctional *SLC26A4* variants as compared to functional null alleles in PDS patients. This hypothesis was not supported by the subsequent association of a variety of EVA mutations with both PDS and NSEVA [43, 49].

Differential effects of mutations on Cl^-/HCO_3^- exchange versus Cl^-/I^- exchange activities similarly lack a clear causal correlation with thyroid phenotype [31, 42]. Another study concluded that the thyroid phenotype, as defined by the perchlorate discharge test, is correlated with the number of *SLC26A4* mutant alleles [9]. By that criterion, PDS is a genetically homogenous disease entity caused by two mutant alleles of *SLC26A4* whereas NSEVA is usually associated with zero or one mutant alleles [9, 50].

Approximately 3/4 of Caucasian EVA patients carry only one or zero mutant alleles of *SLC26A4* [9, 10, 31, 47, 51, 52]. The detection of only one mutant allele of *SLC26A4* in an EVA patient is non-diagnostic, and potential misclassification of hypofunctional variants such as p.R776C further contributes to diagnostic uncertainty [31, 53]. If a *SLC26A4* variant is usually or always detected as the sole variant in NSEVA patients, then the variant may be coincidental and non-pathogenic [31]. Alternatively, a single pathogenic mutation of *SLC26A4* is likely to cause EVA in combination with a second occult mutation of *SLC26A4* (DFNB4) or, less likely, another autosomal gene [9, 12, 47, 54]. Rare heterozygous, hypomorphic missense variants of *FOXI1* [55] and *KCNJ10* [56] were proposed to cause EVA as a digenic trait in combination with a heterozygous *SLC26A4* mutation. However, this conclusion has not been supported by other studies [57], and the published data do not exclude alternative interpretations [58].

Thyroid and auditory phenotypes in EVA patients with one mutant allele are usually, if not always, less severe than those in patients with two mutant alleles of *SLC26A4* [9, 22, 28, 59]. Unilateral EVA is more prevalent among EVA patients with zero or one mutant allele, whereas patients with two mutant alleles of *SLC26A4* usually have bilateral EVA [9, 47, 59].

EVA in patients with no detectable *SLC26A4* mutations appears to be caused by non-genetic factors, by mutations in other genes, or by both as part of a complex trait, as evidenced by low recurrence risk and discordant segregation of EVA with *SLC26A4* [12, 47, 51]. However, specific non-genetic causes have not yet been identified [60].

Diagnosis

PDS is now usually detected by the identification of EVA in temporal bone imaging studies of children with sensorineural hearing loss. A comprehensive medical history and physical examination should be performed to identify other causes of deafness. The detection of two mutant alleles of *SLC26A4* provides a conclusive molecular genetic diagnosis. A perchlorate discharge test is appropriate in cases with non-diagnostic *SLC26A4* genotypes (i.e. one or zero detectable mutations), goiter, or both [28]. Cases with a clinically normal thyroid, non-diagnostic *SLC26A4* genotype, but a positive perchlorate discharge result warrant surveillance of the thyroid.

Management

Conventional hearing amplification is adequate in many cases with significant residual hearing. Patients with residual hearing should be counseled to avoid head trauma, since even mild head trauma or barotrauma can cause sudden hearing loss in some patients. When hearing loss is profound, cochlear implantation can be considered. Many EVA patients, irrespective of the presence of a cochlear anomaly, have undergone cochlear implantation with functional results comparable to those in children with no cochleovestibular anomalies [61, 62]. Perilymph leakage may be observed during cochleostomy in patients with incomplete partition, but is usually self-limited or easily controlled [61–63].

Management of the thyroid gland includes surveillance and treatment for goiter and, in some cases, functional hypothyroidism. Hypothyroidism typically affects individuals with a large or long-standing goiter. Since both penetrance and prevalence of goiter exceed those of hypothyroidism, surveillance of thyroid volume is recommended in patients with iodide organification defects. This is best achieved with periodic ultrasound evaluations. Levothyroxine has been used to prevent or retard progression or symptoms of goiter, although efficacy of this practice has not been tested by rigorous clinical trial. Subtotal thyroidectomy may be necessary in extreme cases. Functional hypothyroidism is uncommon, and should be treated with levothyroxine.

Conclusion

Recent advances in molecular genetics and clinical evaluation have transformed the detection and diagnosis of PDS. The diagnosis is confirmed by detection of two mutant alleles of *SLC26A4* in a patient with EVA. The perchlorate discharge test can detect the underlying thyroid biochemical defect and is useful for the evaluation of goiter or for supporting the diagnosis of PDS in a patient with a non-diagnostic *SLC26A4* genotype. Treatment is focused upon rehabilitation of hearing loss, and surveillance and management of goiter and, less commonly, hypothyroidism. An *Slc26a4*$^{\Delta}$ (knockout) mouse model facilitates investigation of this disorder, but the mechanism of hearing loss remains unclear.

References

1 Brucker-Davis F, Skarulis MC, Pikus A, Ishizawar D, Mastroianni MA, Koby M, Weintraub BD: Prevalence and mechanisms of hearing loss in patients with resistance to thyroid hormone. J Clin Endocrinol Metab 1996;81:2768–2772.
2 Pendred V: Deaf-mutism and goitre. Lancet 1896;ii:532.
3 Morgans ME, Trotter WR: Association of congenital deafness with goitre; the nature of the thyroid defect. Lancet 1958;i:607–609.
4 Phelps PD, Coffey RA, Trembath RC, et al: Radiological malformations of the ear in Pendred syndrome. Clin Radiol 1998; 53:268–273.
5 Fraser GR: Association of congenital deafness with goitre (Pendred's syndrome) a study of 207 families. Ann Hum Genet 1965;28:201–249.
6 Everett LA, Glaser B, Beck JC, et al: Pendred syndrome is caused by mutations in a putative sulphate transporter gene (PDS). Nat Genet 1997;17:411–422.
7 Li XC, Everett LA, Lalwani AK, Desmukh D, Friedman TB, Green ED, Wilcox ER: A mutation in PDS causes non-syndromic recessive deafness. Nat Genet 1998;18:215–217.
8 Usami S, Abe S, Weston MD, Shinkawa H, Van Camp G, Kimberling WJ: Non-syndromic hearing loss associated with enlarged vestibular aqueduct is caused by PDS mutations. Hum Genet 1999; 104:188–192.
9 Pryor SP, Madeo AC, Reynolds JC, et al: SLC26A4/PDS genotype-phenotype correlation in hearing loss with enlargement of the vestibular aqueduct (EVA): evidence that Pendred syndrome and non-syndromic EVA are distinct clinical and genetic entities. J Med Genet 2005; 42:159–165.
10 Albert S, Blons H, Jonard L, et al: SLC26A4 gene is frequently involved in nonsyndromic hearing impairment with enlarged vestibular aqueduct in Caucasian populations. Eur J Hum Genet 2006;14:773–779.
11 Birkenhager R, Zimmer AJ, Maier W, Klenzner T, Aschendorff A, Schipper J: Evidence of a novel gene for the LAV-syndrome. Laryngo-Rhino-Otologie 2007;86:102–106.
12 Choi BY, Madeo AC, King KA, Zalewski CK, Pryor SP, Muskett JA, Nance WE, Butman JA, Brewer CC, Griffith AJ: Segregation of enlarged vestibular aqueducts in families with non-diagnostic SLC26A4 genotypes. J Med Genet 2009; 46:856–861.
13 Anwar S, Riazuddin S, Ahmed ZM, Tasneem S, Ateeq ul J, Khan SY, Griffith AJ, Friedman TB, Riazuddin S: SLC26A4 mutation spectrum associated with DFNB4 deafness and Pendred's syndrome in Pakistanis. J Hum Genet 2009; 54:266–270.
14 Fraser GR: Deafness with goiter (Pendred's syndrome). Baltimore, Johns Hopkins University Press, 1976.
15 Park HJ, Shaukat S, Liu XZ, et al: Origins and frequencies of SLC26A4 (PDS) mutations in east and south Asians: global implications for the epidemiology of deafness. J Med Genet 2003;40:242–248.
16 Stinckens C, Huygen PL, Joosten FB, Van Camp G, Otten B, Cremers CW: Fluctuant, progressive hearing loss associated with Meniere like vertigo in three patients with the Pendred syndrome. Int J Pediatr Otorhinolaryngol 2001;61:207–215.
17 Valvassori GE, Clemis JD: The large vestibular aqueduct syndrome. Laryngoscope 1978;88:723–728.
18 Govaerts PJ, Casselman J, Daemers K, De Ceulaer G, Somers T, Offeciers FE: Audiological findings in large vestibular aqueduct syndrome. Int J Pediatr Otorhinolaryngol 1999;51:157–164.

19 Nakashima T, Ueda H, Furuhashi A, Sato E, Asahi K, Naganawa S, Beppu R: Air-bone gap and resonant frequency in large vestibular aqueduct syndrome. Am J Otol 2000;21:671–674.
20 Arjmand EM, Webber A: Audiometric findings in children with a large vestibular aqueduct. Arch Otolaryngol Head Neck Surg 2004;130:1169–1174.
21 Merchant SN, Nakajima HH, Halpin C, Nadol JB Jr, Lee DJ, Innis WP, Curtin H, Rosowski JJ: Clinical investigation and mechanism of air-bone gaps in large vestibular aqueduct syndrome. Ann Otol Rhinol Laryngol 2007;116:532–541.
22 King KA, Choi BY, Zalewski C, et al: SLC26A4 genotype, but not cochlear radiologic structure, is correlated with hearing loss in ears with an enlarged vestibular aqueduct. Laryngoscope 2010;120:384–389.
23 Zhou G, Gopen Q, Kenna MA: Delineating the hearing loss in children with enlarged vestibular aqueduct. Laryngoscope 2008;118:2062–2066.
24 Hvidberg-Hansen J, Jorgensen MB: The inner ear in Pendred's syndrome. Acta Oto-Laryngol 1968;66:129–135.
25 Choi BY, Stewart AK, Nishimura KK, et al: Efficient molecular genetic diagnosis of enlarged vestibular aqueducts in East Asians. Genet Testing Mol Biomarkers 2009;13:679–687.
26 Colvin IB, Beale T, Harrop-Griffiths K: Long-term follow-up of hearing loss in children and young adults with enlarged vestibular aqueducts: relationship to radiologic findings and Pendred syndrome diagnosis. Laryngoscope 2006;116:2027–2036.
27 Reardon W, Coffey R, Phelps PD, Luxon LM, Stephens D, Kendall-Taylor P, Britton KE, Grossman A, Trembath R: Pendred syndrome – 100 years of underascertainment? Q J Med 1997;90:443–447.
28 Madeo AC, Manichaikul A, Reynolds JC, Sarlis NJ, Pryor SP, Shawker TH, Griffith AJ: Evaluation of the thyroid in patients with hearing loss and enlarged vestibular aqueducts. Arch Otolaryngol Head Neck Surg 2009;135:670–676.
29 Reardon W, Coffey R, Chowdhury T, Grossman A, Jan H, Britton K, Kendall-Taylor P, Trembath R: Prevalence, age of onset, and natural history of thyroid disease in Pendred syndrome. J Med Genet 1999;36:595–598.
30 Johnsen T, Larsen C, Friis J, Hougaard-Jensen F: Pendred's syndrome: acoustic, vestibular and radiological findings in 17 unrelated patients. J Laryngol Otol 1987;101:1187–1192.
31 Choi BY, Stewart AK, Madeo AC, et al: Hypo-functional SLC26A4 variants associated with nonsyndromic hearing loss and enlargement of the vestibular aqueduct: genotype-phenotype correlation or coincidental polymorphisms? Hum Mutat 2009;30:599–608.
32 Scott DA, Wang R, Kreman TM, Sheffield VC, Karniski LP: The Pendred syndrome gene encodes a chloride-iodide transport protein. Nat Genet 1999;21:440–443.
33 Scott DA, Karniski LP: Human pendrin expressed in *Xenopus laevis* oocytes mediates chloride/formate exchange. Am J Physiol 2000;278:C207–C211.
34 Royaux IE, Wall SM, Karniski LP, Everett LA, Suzuki K, Knepper MA, Green ED: Pendrin, encoded by the Pendred syndrome gene, resides in the apical region of renal intercalated cells and mediates bicarbonate secretion. Proc Natl Acad Sci USA 2001;98:4221–4226.
35 Gillam MP, Sidhaye AR, Lee EJ, Rutishauser J, Stephan CW, Kopp P: Functional characterization of pendrin in a polarized cell system: evidence for pendrin-mediated apical iodide efflux. J Biol Chem 2004;279:13004–13010.
36 Royaux IE, Belyantseva IA, Wu T, Kachar B, Everett LA, Marcus DC, Green ED: Localization and functional studies of pendrin in the mouse inner ear provide insight about the etiology of deafness in pendred syndrome. J Assoc Res Otolaryngol 2003;4:394–404.
37 Everett LA, Belyantseva IA, Noben-Trauth K, Cantos R, Chen A, Thakkar SI, Hoogstraten-Miller SL, Kachar B, Wu DK, Green ED: Targeted disruption of mouse PDS provides insight about the inner-ear defects encountered in Pendred syndrome. Hum Mol Genet 2001;10:153–161.
38 Jabba SV, Oelke A, Singh R, Maganti RJ, Fleming S, Wall SM, Everett LA, Green ED, Wangemann P: Macrophage invasion contributes to degeneration of stria vascularis in Pendred syndrome mouse model. BMC Med 2006;4:37.
39 Wangemann P, Nakaya K, Wu T, Maganti RJ, Itza EM, Sanneman JD, Harbidge DG, Billings S, Marcus DC: Loss of cochlear HCO_3^- secretion causes deafness via endolymphatic acidification and inhibition of Ca^{2+} reabsorption in a Pendred syndrome mouse model. Am J Physiol Renal Physiol 2007;292:F1345–F1353.
40 Singh R, Wangemann P: Free radical stress-mediated loss of Kcnj10 protein expression in stria vascularis contributes to deafness in Pendred syndrome mouse model. Am J Physiol Renal Physiol 2008; 294:F139–F148.
41 Wangemann P, Kim HM, Billings S, Nakaya K, Li X, Singh R, Sharlin DS, Forrest D, Marcus DC, Fong P: Developmental delays consistent with cochlear hypothyroidism contribute to failure to develop hearing in mice lacking Slc26a4/pendrin expression. Am J Physiol Renal Physiol 2009;297: F1435–F1447.
42 Dai P, Stewart AK, Chebib F, et al: Distinct and novel SLC26A4/Pendrin mutations in Chinese and US patients with nonsyndromic hearing loss. Physiol Genom 2009;38:281–290.
43 Tsukamoto K, Suzuki H, Harada D, Namba A, Abe S, Usami S: Distribution and frequencies of PDS (SLC26A4) mutations in Pendred syndrome and nonsyndromic hearing loss associated with enlarged vestibular aqueduct: a unique spectrum of mutations in Japanese. Eur J Hum Genet 2003; 11:916–922.
44 Wu CC, Yeh TH, Chen PJ, Hsu CJ: Prevalent SLC26A4 mutations in patients with enlarged vestibular aqueduct and/or Mondini dysplasia: a unique spectrum of mutations in Taiwan, including a frequent founder mutation. Laryngoscope 2005;115:1060–1064.
45 Park HJ, Lee SJ, Jin HS, et al: Genetic basis of hearing loss associated with enlarged vestibular aqueducts in Koreans. Clin Genet 2005;67:160–165.
46 Dai P, Li Q, Huang D, et al: SLC26A4 c.919–2A>G varies among Chinese ethnic groups as a cause of hearing loss. Genet Med 2008;10:586–592.
47 Azaiez H, Yang T, Prasad S, Sorensen JL, Nishimura CJ, Kimberling WJ, Smith RJ: Genotype-phenotype correlations for SLC26A4-related deafness. Hum Genet 2007;122:451–457.

48 Scott DA, Wang R, Kreman TM, Andrews M, McDonald JM, Bishop JR, Smith RJH, Karniski LP, Sheffield VC: Functional differences of the *PDS* gene product are associated with phenotypic variation in patients with Pendred syndrome and non-syndromic hearing loss (DFNB4). Hum Mol Genet 2000;9:1709–1715.

49 Lopez-Bigas N, Melchionda S, de Cid R, Grifa A, Zelante L, Govea N, Arbones ML, Gasparini P, Estivill X: Identification of five new mutations of PDS/SLC26A4 in Mediterranean families with hearing impairment. Hum Mutat 2001;18:548.

50 Pera A, Dossena S, Rodighiero S, Gandia M, Botta G, Meyer G, Moreno F, Nofziger C, Hernandez-Chico C, Paulmichl M: Functional assessment of allelic variants in the SLC26A4 gene involved in Pendred syndrome and nonsyndromic EVA. Proc Natl Acad Sci USA 2008;105:18608–18613.

51 Campbell C, Cucci RA, Prasad S, Green GE, Edeal JB, Galer CE, Karniski LP, Sheffield VC, Smith RJ: Pendred syndrome, DFNB4, and PDS/SLC26A4 identification of eight novel mutations and possible genotype-phenotype correlations. Hum Mutat 2001;17:403–411.

52 Pera A, Villamar M, Vinuela A, Gandia M, Meda C, Moreno F, Hernandez-Chico C: A mutational analysis of the SLC26A4 gene in Spanish hearing-impaired families provides new insights into the genetic causes of Pendred syndrome and DFNB4 hearing loss. Eur J Hum Genet 2008;16:888–896.

53 Pfarr N, Borck G, Turk A, Napiontek U, Keilmann A, Muller-Forell W, Kopp P, Pohlenz J: Goitrous congenital hypothyroidism and hearing impairment associated with mutations in the TPO and SLC26A4/PDS genes. J Clin Endocrinol Metab 2006;91:2678–2681.

54 Kimberling WJ: Estimation of the frequency of occult mutations for an autosomal recessive disease in the presence of genetic heterogeneity: application to genetic hearing loss disorders. Hum Mutat 2005;26:462–470.

55 Yang T, Vidarsson H, Rodrigo-Blomqvist S, Rosengren SS, Enerback S, Smith RJ: Transcriptional control of SLC26A4 is involved in Pendred syndrome and nonsyndromic enlargement of vestibular aqueduct (DFNB4). Am J Hum Genet 2007;80:1055–1063.

56 Yang T, Gurrola JG 2nd, Wu H, Chiu SM, Wangemann P, Snyder PM, Smith RJ: Mutations of KCNJ10 together with mutations of SLC26A4 cause digenic nonsyndromic hearing loss associated with enlarged vestibular aqueduct syndrome. Am J Hum Genet 2009;84:651–657.

57 Wu CC, Lu YC, Chen PJ, Yeh PL, Su YN, Hwu WL, Hsu CJ: Phenotypic analyses and mutation screening of the SLC26A4 and FOXI1 genes in 101 Taiwanese families with bilateral nonsyndromic enlarged vestibular aqueduct (DFNB4) or Pendred syndrome. Audiol Neuro-Otol 2009;15:57–66.

58 Choi BY, Alper SL, Griffith AJ: Response to: The c.-103T>C variant in the 5′-UTR of SLC26A4 gene: a pathogenic mutation or coincidental polymorphism? Reply to Yang T, et al. [letter]. Hum Mutat 2009;30:1471. Included with PubMed PMID 19787632.

59 Madden C, Halsted M, Meinzen-Derr J, et al: The influence of mutations in the SLC26A4 gene on the temporal bone in a population with enlarged vestibular aqueduct. Arch Otolar Head Neck Surg 2007;133:162–168.

60 Pryor SP, Demmler GJ, Madeo AC, Yang Y, Zalewski CK, Brewer CC, Butman JA, Fowler KB, Griffith AJ: Investigation of the role of congenital cytomegalovirus infection in the etiology of enlarged vestibular aqueducts. Arch Otolar Head Neck Surg 2005;131:388–392.

61 Loundon N, Rouillon I, Munier N, Marlin S, Roger G, Garabedian EN: Cochlear implantation in children with internal ear malformations. Otol Neurotol 2005;26:668–673.

62 Papsin BC: Cochlear implantation in children with anomalous cochleovestibular anatomy. Laryngoscope 2005;115(suppl 106):1–26.

63 Aschendorff A, Marangos N, Laszig R: Large vestibular aqueduct syndrome and its implication for cochlear implant surgery. Am J Otol 1997;18(suppl 6):S57.

Dr. A.J. Griffith
5 Research Court, Room 2B-28
Rockville, MD 20850 (USA)
Tel. +1 301 496 1960, Fax +1 301 402 7580, E-Mail griffita@nidcd.nih.gov

Alford RL, Sutton VR (eds): Medical Genetics in the Clinical Practice of ORL.
Adv Otorhinolaryngol. Basel, Karger, 2011, vol 70, pp 50–55

Pigmentary Anomalies and Hearing Loss

Helga V. Toriello

Genetics Services, Spectrum Health Hospitals, and College of Human Medicine, Michigan State University, Grand Rapids, Mich., USA

Abstract

A number of syndromes that include hearing loss in the phenotype also have pigmentary anomalies as a component manifestation. One of the most common of these is Waardenburg syndrome, which includes hypopigmentation and sensorineural hearing loss in the phenotype. There are four types of Waardenburg syndrome, distinguishable from each other by clinical findings. However, there are several other syndromes which include not only hypopigmentation, but also hyperpigmentation in the phenotype. This paper serves as a review of many of these syndromes.

It is not unusual to find the combination of pigmentary abnormalities and hearing loss occurring together, either as component manifestations of a syndrome such as Waardenburg syndrome, or as an association, as is the case in vitiligo. One reason for this co-occurrence is that melanocytes are involved in both pigmentation and as components of the inner ear. Melanocytes arise from the neural crest precursor cells called melanoblasts. These cells migrate to their final sites which are the skin; hair bulb; uveal tract of the eye; stria vascularis, vestibular organ, and endolymphatic sac of the ear; and leptomeninges of the brain. Development of melanocytes from the neural crest and migration to these sites are regulated by a signaling pathway which includes several relevant genes, including *PAX3*, *MITF*, *SOX10*, *KIT*, *EDN3*, *EDNBB*, and *SNAI2* (see review by Sato-Jin et al. [1]). Other genes are needed for post-migrational function, but mutations in few, if any, are associated with hearing loss [2].

Hypopigmenation Syndromes

Waardenburg Syndromes

One of the most common groups of syndromes which have the occurrence of both pigmentary anomalies and hearing loss is the various forms of Waardenburg syndrome. In a recent survey of 1,763 individuals with hearing loss, Tamayo et al. [3] found that one of the Waardenburg syndromes (types I and II) accounted for 5.38% of the cases. This is a heterogeneous group of conditions, which were first classified on a clinical basis. There are four main types, called Waardenburg types I–IV. Waardenburg syndrome type I (WS1) is characterized by pigmentary anomalies, including frontal white forelock, premature graying of the hair, 2 different colored eyes or partially colored iris of one eye, and/or bright blue irides. Craniofacial features are distinctive, and include lateral displacement of the inner canthi, synophrys, and broad and high nasal root with hypoplastic alae nasi. The Waardenburg Consortium [4] has proposed diagnostic criteria for the diagnosis of WS1. In order to be considered affected, an individual needs to have two major or one major plus two minor criteria. Major criteria include congenital sensorineural hearing loss, pigmentary disturbances of the iris, white forelock, dystopia canthorum, with a W index above 1.95, and affected first degree relative. The W index is calculated by measuring the inner canthal distance (a), the interpupillary distance (b), and the outer canthal distance (c). Using these figures, calculate X ((2a–.2119c–3.909)/c) and Y ((2a–.2479b–3.9.9)/b). The W index is X + Y + a/b. For example, if an individual has an inner canthal distance of 35 mm, an interpupillary distance of 60 mm, and an outer canthal distance of 90 mm, the W index would be approximately 1.96 indicating dystopia canthorum. Minor criteria include several areas of hypopigmented skin, synophrys or medial eyebrow flare, broad and high nasal root, hypoplastic alae nasi, and premature graying of hair, with the head hair predominantly white by the age of 30 years [4].

Waardenburg syndrome type II (WS2) is distinguished from WS1 by the absence of craniofacial anomalies, particularly the lack of dystopia canthorum (and thus a W index of less than 1.95). The pigmentary anomalies are similar to those of WS1, and include white forelock, depigmented skin patches, and heterochromia. Diagnostic criteria proposed for type II require that 2 of 4 major findings be present in an individual, with those findings including congenital sensorineural hearing loss, pigmentary disturbance of the iris, pigmentary disturbance of the hair, and an affected first degree relative [5]. An additional clinical distinction between the two forms is that congenital hearing loss tends to occur more frequently in WS2 than it does in WS1, with recent reports suggesting that hearing loss occurs in up to 75% of those with WS1, and up to 91% of those with WS2 [6]. The degree of loss is highly variable, ranging from mild, unilateral hearing loss to severe congenital bilateral sensorineural hearing loss. In addition, one group found that most individuals with WS1 and WS2 have vestibular disturbances, even if hearing is normal [7]. It was recommended that electrocochleography and vestibular function testing be done in all individuals with WS.

Waardenburg syndrome type III (WS3) is also called Klein-Waardenburg syndrome. Individuals with this form of WS have in addition to hearing loss, pigmentary anomalies, and craniofacial manifestations; musculoskeletal anomalies of the upper limbs. These anomalies range from severe hypoplasia of the limb to flexion contractures of the digits [8, 9].

Waardenburg syndrome type IV (WS4) is also termed Waardenburg-Shah syndrome, and is characterized by the additional finding of Hirschsprung disease. Hearing loss occurs less frequently in this type of WS, being reported in only 5% in one study [10]. A subtype of WS4 has also been described. In this form, a peripheral demyelinating neuropathy as well as central dysmyelination also occurs in addition to Waardenburg manifestations and Hirschsprung disease. This condition is also known as PCWH (peripheral demyelinating neuropathy, central dysmyelination, Waardenburg syndrome, and Hirschsprung disease) [11, 12]. It is noteworthy, however, that Hirschsprung disease does not always occur in individuals considered to have this condition [13].

Given the phenotypic overlap of these conditions, it should not be a surprise that mutations in genes with related function are the cause of these entities. Heterozygous mutations in *PAX3* are responsible for causing Waardenburg syndrome type I, as well as some cases of Waardenburg syndrome type III. In addition, homozygous mutations in *PAX3* have been reported to be responsible for at least one case of WS3. WS2 can be caused by mutations in several genes, including *MITF*, *SOX10*, *SNAI2*, as well as two as yet to be identified genes that map to 1p and 8p23. WS2 caused by *MITF* or *SOX10* mutation is inherited as an autosomal dominant condition; those caused by mutations in *SNAI2* are inherited in an autosomal recessive fashion. WS4 is also heterogeneous, and

Table 1. Waardenburg syndromes and molecular causes

Type of Waardenburg syndrome	Gene	Mode of inheritance
Waardenburg type I	*PAX3*	AD
Waardenburg type II	*MITF*	AD
	SNAI2	AR
	SOX10	AD
	unknown	AD
Waardenburg type III	*PAX3*	AD, AR
Waardenburg type IV	*EDNRB*	AD, AR
	EDN3	AD, AR
	SOX10	AD
Craniofacial-deafness-hand syndrome	*PAX3*	AD
	unknown	
Tietz-Smith syndrome	*MITF*	AD
ABCD syndrome	*EDNRB*	AR
Yemenite deaf-blind syndrome	*SOX10*	AD
	unknown	

AD = autosomal-dominant; AR = autosomal-recessive.

can be caused by heterozygous or homozygous mutations in *EDNRB* or *EDN3*, or heterozygous mutations in SOX10. In addition, heterozygous mutations in *SOX10* cause *PCWH*, the neurologic variant of WS4 (table 1).

Waardenburg-Related Conditions

There are also a few conditions that were initially considered to be unique entities, but that have subsequently been found to be caused by mutations in some of the above-mentioned genes. The craniofacial-deafness-hand syndrome (CDHS) was first described by Sommer et al. [14] in 1983. The phenotype consists of severe sensorineural hearing loss, flat facial profile, hypertelorism, downslanting palpebral fissures, depressed nasal bridge, small mouth, and ulnar deviation and contractures of the hands. Radiographs have found hypoplasia of the nasal bones and ulnar styloid. A similarly affected individual was reported by Gad et al. [15]. However, the patients reported by Sommer et al. were subsequently found to have mutation of *PAX3*, making this condition allelic to WS1 [16]. Gad et al.'s patient had gene sequencing of *PAX3*, with no pathologic alteration found, thus indicating that there is apparent causal heterogeneity in CDHS.

Tietz-Smith syndrome is an autosomal dominant condition characterized by oculocutaneous albinism and profound congenital sensorineural hearing loss. The degree of hearing loss is at least 100 dB. The albinism is limited to skin and hair, although darkening of the skin and hair can occur with age. The irides are described as being normal; the fundus may also be normal or demonstrate mild albinoid changes [17]. Mutation in the *MITF* gene has been found to cause this syndrome, thus it is allelic to WS2 [18].

The Yemenite deaf-blind syndrome is a rare condition characterized by hypopigmentation of skin and hair, ocular abnormalities (including microcornea, coloboma, and/or visual impairment). Hearing loss is congenital and sensorineural, but may also have a conductive component [19]. This is likely heterogeneous; one individual was found to have a heterozygous *SOX10* mutation, whereas a pair of siblings did not have mutations in *SOX10* [19, 20].

The ABCD syndrome is an autosomal-recessive condition characterized by albinism, black hair lock(s), cell migration disorder of neurocytes (i.e. Hirschsprung disease), and deafness. Affected individuals also have retinal depigmentation. The eyelashes and eyebrows are white, and the irides bright blue. ABCD syndrome has only been reported in one consanguineous family. Cause of this condition is homozygous mutation in the *EDNRB* gene, which is one of the genes that can cause WS4. It is noteworthy that heterozygous carriers had no clinical manifestations [21].

Other Conditions with Hypopigmentation and Hearing Loss

There are a few other conditions in which the combination of hypopigmentation and hearing loss occurs. All of these conditions are rare, having been reported in only one or two families or individuals.

Tak et al. [22] reported on a female patient with ocular albinism with sensorineural deafness. Her father and brother reportedly had the same manifestations. In addition to ocular albinism, the irides were reported to be blue (which were unusual for her ethnic background), and multiple pigmented lentigenes were present on her face and upper limbs. A similar family had been reported by Bard [23]; this family was subsequently found to have heterozygous mutations in *MITF*, as well as homozygous or heterozygous polymorphisms of the tyrosinase gene (Tyr, which is regulated by *MITF*). Morrell et al. [24], who described the molecular findings in this family, postulated that digenic inheritance is responsible for the combination of a WS phenotype with ocular albinism. However, no molecular studies were done on the family reported by Tak et al. [22], so the possibility that heterogeneity exists certainly cannot be ruled out.

Ziprkowski et al. [25] and Margolis [26] described an X-linked pedigree in which the individuals had hypopigmented skin at birth (the only exception was lightly pigmented skin on the lower trunk) and congenital profound sensorineural hearing loss. Over time, pigmentation gradually increased, leading to areas of hyperpigmentation, particularly affecting the lower trunk, but also affecting limbs and face. However, the hair, which was white at birth, remained unpigmented, even if growing in a pigmented area of skin. There has been the suggestion that the condition reported by Woolf et al. [27] in two boys is the same as this entity. The latter two boys also had congenital sensorineural hearing loss, but had a different pattern of pigmentation. In these two boys the head, hair, and upper chest were depigmented, whereas the remainder of their bodies had normal pigmentation. This question remains unresolved, since the molecular defect has not been found in either family.

There is also a report of a single individual with piebaldism and profound congenital hearing loss. A heterozygous mutation in the *KIT* proto-oncogene was found in this individual. It is possible that the occurrence of hearing loss in those with piebaldism is mutation-specific, since those with piebaldism generally do not have hearing loss [28].

Hyperpigmentation Disorders

Leopard Syndrome

Perhaps one of the most common conditions in which hyperpigmentation and hearing loss both occur is the so-called LEOPARD syndrome. This syndrome name is an acronym for lentigines (multiple), electrocardiographic defects, ocular hypertelorism, pulmonary stenosis, abnormalities of genitalia, retardation of growth, and sensorineural deafness. The lentigines (which resemble freckles but are histologically distinct from them) can be present at birth, but more often appear during early childhood, increasing in number during puberty. Electrocardiographic defects are present in approximately 75%, and pulmonary stenosis affects 10–20%. Hypertrophic cardiomyopathy is also a fairly common finding, and often manifests before the development of the lentigines [29]. Genital anomalies are more apparent in males, with cryptorchidism present in at least half; hypospadias and genital hypoplasia also occur. In females, delayed puberty and ovarian hypoplasia are most common. Sensorineural hearing loss affects 15–25%, and can be congenital, but also develop later in life. The facial phenotype is characteristic, and in addition to including hypertelorism, also can include ptosis, flat nasal bridge, thick lips, and dysmorphic ears. LEOPARD syndrome is heterogeneous, with mutations in three different genes identified to date. The most common genetic cause is heterozygous mutation in the *PTPN11* gene, which is also responsible for about 50% of cases of Noonan syndrome. In addition, heterozygous mutations in *RAF1* (which can also be mutated in a small portion of individuals with Noonan syndrome) and *BRAF* (which is mutated in the majority of individuals with cardiofaciocutaneous syndrome) have also been reported to occur in those with the clinical diagnosis of LEOPARD syndrome [29, 30].

H Syndrome
The H syndrome is a recently described autosomal-recessive syndrome with numerous manifestations, including hyperpigmentation, hypertrichosis, hepatosplenomegaly, heart anomalies, hearing loss, hypogonadism, low height (short stature), and hyperglycemia. Skin findings are characterized by hyperpigmentation and hypertrichotic lesions which develop during the third and fourth decade of life. These lesions are primarily on the lower half of the body. Cardiac anomalies include pulmonic stenosis, patent ductus arteriosus, or murmur. In females, hypogonadism manifests as delayed puberty and amenorrhea; in males, micropenis is the more common finding. Diabetes is present in approximately 20%, but may be the first manifestation of the syndrome [31].

Additional physical manifestations include hallux valgus and flexion contractures of the proximal interphalangeal joints, facial telangiectasias, and arcus senilis. The hearing loss, which is sensorineural, is not present in all with this syndrome. The cause of this condition was recently discovered to be homozygous mutation in the *SLC29A3* gene, whose function is as a nucleoside transporter [32, 33].

References

1 Sato-Jin K, Nishimura EK, Akasaka E, Huber W, Nakano H, Miller A, Du J, Wu M, Hanada K, Sawamura D, Fisher DE, Imokawa G: Epistatic connections between microphthalmia-associated transcription factor and endothelin signaling in Waardenburg syndrome and other pigmentary disorders. FASEB J 2008;22:1155–1168.
2 Dessinioti C, Stratigos AJ, Rigopoulos D, Katsambas AD: A review of genetic disorders of hypopigmentation: lessons learned from the biology of melanocytes. Dermatol 2009;18:741–749.
3 Tamayo ML, Gelvez N, Rodriguez M, Florez S, Varon C, Medina D, Bernal JE: Screening program for Waardenburg syndrome in Colombia: clinical definition and phenotypic variability. Am J Med Genet Pt. A 2008;146A:1026–1031.
4 Read AP, Newton VE: Waardenburg syndrome. J Med Genet 1997;34:656–665.
5 Liu XZ, Newton VE, Read AP: Waardenburg syndrome type 2: phenotypic findings and diagnostic criteria. Am J Med Genet 1995;55:95–100.
6 Oysu C, Baserer N, Tinaz M: Audiometric manifestations of Waardenburg's syndrome. Ear Nose Throat J 2000;79:704–709.
7 Black FO, Pesznecker SC, Allen K, Gianna C: A vestibular phenotype for Waardenburg syndrome? Otol Neurotol 2001;22:188–194.
8 Goodman RM, Lewithal I, Solomon A, Klein D: Upper limb involvement in the Klein-Waardenburg syndrome. Am J Med Genet 1982;11:425–433.
9 Wollnik B, Tukel T, Uyguner O, Ghanbari A, Kayserili H, Emiroglu M, Yuksel-Apak M: Homozygous and heterozygous inheritance of PAX3 mutations causes different types of Waardenburg syndrome. Am J Med Genet 2003; 122A:42–45.
10 Puffenberger EG, Hosoda K, Washington SS, Nakao K, deWit D, Tanagisawa M, Chakravarti A: A missense mutation of the endothelin-B receptor gene in multigenic Hirschsprung's disease. Cell 1994; 79:1257–1266.
11 Pingault V, Guiochon-Mantel A, Bondurand N, Faure C, Lacroix C, Lyonnet S, Goossens M, Landrieu P: Peripheral neuropathy with hypomyelination, chronic intestinal pseudo-obstruction and deafness: a developmental 'neural crest syndrome' related to a SOX10 mutation. Ann Neurol 2000;48: 671–676.
12 Inoue K, Shilo K, Boerkoel CF, Crowe C, Sawady J, Lupski JR, Agamanolis DP: Congenital hypomyelinating neuropathy, central dysmyelination, and Waardenburg-Hirschsprung disease: phenotypes linked by SOX10 mutation. Ann Neurol 2002;52:836–842.

13 Sznajer Y, Coldea C, Meire F, Delpierre I, Sekhara T, Touraine RL: A de novo SOX10 mutation causing severe type 4 Waardenburg syndrome without Hirschsprung disease. Am J Med Genet 2008;146A:1038–1041.
14 Sommer A, Young-Wee T, Frye T: Previously undescribed syndrome of craniofacial, hand anomalies, and sensorineural deafness. Am J Med Genet 1983;15:71–77.
15 Gad A, Laurino M, Maravilla KR, Matsushita M, Raskind WH: Sensorineural deafness, distinctive facial features, and abnormal cranial bones: a new variant of Waardenburg syndrome? Am J Med Genet Pt. A 2008; 146A:1880–1885.
16 Asher JJ, Sommer A, Morell R, Friedman T: Missense mutation in the paired domain of PAX3 causes craniofacial-deafness-hand syndrome. Hum Mutat 1996;7:30–35.
17 Smith SD, Kelley PM, Kenyon JB, Hoover D: Tietz syndrome (hypopigmentation/deafness) caused by mutation of MITF. J Med Genet 2000;37:446–448.
18 Izumi K, Kohta T, Kimura Y, Ishida S, Takahashi T, Ishiko A, Kosaki K: Tietz syndrome: unique phenotype specific to mutations of MITF nuclear localization signal. Clin Genet 2008;74:93–95.
19 Warburg M, Tommerup N, Vestermark S, Parving A, Weismann K, Russell B, Thomsen HK: The Yemenite deaf-blind hypopigmentation syndrome. Ophthalmic Paediatr Genet 1990;11: 201–207.
20 Bondurand N, Kuhlbrodt K, Pingault V, Enderich J, Sajus M, Tommerup N, Warburg M, Hennekam RC, Read AP, Wegner M, Goossens M: SOX10 mutation in a mild form of the Yemenite deaf-blind hypopigmentation syndrome. Eur J Hum Genet 1999;7(suppl):95.
21 Verheij JBGM, Kunze J, Osinga J, van Essen AJ, Hofstra RMW: ABCD syndrome is caused by a homozygous mutation in the EDNRB gene. Am J Med Genet 2002;108:223–225.
22 Tak W-J, Kim M-N, Hong C-K, Ro B-I, Song K-Y, Seo S-J: Ocular albinism with sensorineural deafness. Int J Dermatol 2004;43:290–292.
23 Bard LA: Heterogeneity in Waardenburg's syndrome: report of a family with ocular albinism. Arch Ophthalmol 1978;85:530–539.
24 Morell R, Spritz RA, Ho L, Pierpont J, Guo W, Friedman TB, Asher JH Jr: Apparent digenic inheritance of Waardenburg syndrome type 2 (WS2) and autosomal recessive ocular albinism (AROA). Hum Molec Genet 1997;6:659–664.
25 Ziprkowski L, Krokowski A, Adam A, Costeff H, Sade J: Partial albinism and deaf-mutism due to a recessive sex-linked gene. Arch Dermatol 1962;85: 530–539.
26 Margolis E: A new hereditary syndrome – sex-linked deaf mutism associated with total albinism. Acta Genet Stat Med 1962;12:12–19.
27 Woolf Cm, Dolowitz DA, Aldous HE: Congenital deafness associated with piebaldness. Arch Otolaryngol 1965;82: 244–250.
28 Spritz RA, Beighton P: Piebaldism with deafness: molecular evidence for an expanded syndrome. Am J Med Genet 1998;75:101–103.
29 Sarkozy A, Digilio MC, Dallapiccola B: Leopard syndrome. Orph J Rare Dis DOI:10.1186/1750-1172-3-13.
30 Sarkozy A, Carta C, Moretti S, et al: Germline BRAF mutations in Noonan, LEOPARD, and cardiofaciocutaneous syndromes: molecular diversity and associated phenotypic spectrum. Hum Mutat 2009;30:695–702.
31 Broshtilova V, Ramot Y, Molho-Pessach V, Zlotogorski A: Diabetes mellitus may be the earliest and sole manifestation of the H syndrome. Diabet Med 2009; 26:1179–1183.
32 Molho-Pessach V, Lerer I, Abeliovich D, Agha Z, Libdeh AA, Broshtilova V, Elpeleg O, Zlotogorski A: The H syndrome is caused by mutations in the nucleoside transporter hENT3. Am J Hum Genet 2008;83:529–534.
33 Molho-Pessach V, Suarez J, Perrin C, Chiaverini C, Doviner V, Tristan-Clavijo E, Colmenero I, Giuliano F, Torrelo A, Zlotogorski A: The H syndrome: two novel mutations affecting the same amino acid residue of hENT3. J Dermatol Sci 2010;57:59–61.

Helga V. Toriello, PhD
Genetics Services, Spectrum Health Hospitals, 25 Michigan St., Suite 2000
Grand Rapids, MI 49503 (USA)
Tel. +1 616 391 2700, E-Mail Helga.toriello@spectrum-health.org

Alford RL, Sutton VR (eds): Medical Genetics in the Clinical Practice of ORL.
Adv Otorhinolaryngol. Basel, Karger, 2011, vol 70, pp 56–65

Usher Syndrome: Hearing Loss with Vision Loss

Thomas B. Friedman[a] · Julie M. Schultz[a] · Zubair M. Ahmed[b] · Ekaterini T. Tsilou[c] · Carmen C. Brewer[d]

[a]Section on Human Genetics, Laboratory of Molecular Genetics, National Institute on Deafness and Other Communication Disorders (NIDCD), National Institutes of Health (NIH), Rockville, Md., [b]Division of Pediatric Ophthalmology, Cincinnati Children's Hospital Research Foundation, and Department of Ophthalmology, University of Cincinnati, Cincinnati, Ohio, [c]Ophthalmic Genetics and Visual Function Branch, National Eye Institute, and [d]Otolaryngology Branch, National Institute on Deafness and Other Communication Disorders, National Institutes of Health, Rockville, Md., USA

Abstract

Usher syndrome (USH) is a clinically heterogeneous condition characterized by sensorineural hearing loss, progressive retinal degeneration, and vestibular dysfunction. A minimum test battery is described as well as additional clinical evaluations that would provide comprehensive testing of hearing, vestibular function, and visual function in USH patients. USH is also genetically heterogeneous. At least nine genes have been identified with mutations that can cause USH. The proteins encoded by these genes are thought to interact with one another to form a network in the sensory cells of the inner ear and retina.

A young hearing-impaired child is assumed to have non-syndromic deafness if there are no other clinically abnormal features. However, for some cases of non-syndromic deafness of uncertain etiology, the underlying cause is Usher syndrome (USH) [1]. Audiologic and ophthalmologic evaluations of such a child may reveal not only hearing loss, but a combination of vestibular and subtle visual abnormalities foreshadowing USH. Although there are numerous human syndromes that involve the combination of hearing and vision loss, USH accounts for the majority of deaf-blind cases. Other such disorders can be found at the Online Mendelian Inheritance of Man (OMIM; http://www.ncbi.nlm.nih.gov/sites/entrez?db = omim) by querying 'hearing loss and vision loss'. It is the combination of hearing, vestibular and retinal findings that distinguishes USH from these other phenotypes. There are noteworthy reviews of USH [2–4] that provide historical perspectives and are complemented by current evaluations of the primary literature on molecular and functional studies of the proteins encoded by USH genes [5, 6]. This chapter focuses on the auditory, vestibular and visual clinical assessment of Usher syndrome and an update on the genotype-phenotype relationships that have emerged in the last few years.

Usher Syndrome

There are three clinical types of USH [7, 8]. All three types are characterized by progressive loss of vision due to retinitis pigmentosa (RP), but are distinguishable by the hearing and vestibular phenotype. USH type 1 (USH1) is the most severe type and is characterized by profound congenital hearing loss, RP and absent vestibular function. A congenitally deaf child who is late in walking independently should raise suspicion of USH1. In contrast, USH2 patients have stable, moderate-to-severe hearing loss, normal vestibular function, and RP, while the USH3 phenotype is characterized by progressive loss of hearing, variable degrees of vestibular dysfunction, and RP with an onset in the second to fourth decades of life. Many USH3 individuals have impaired but useful vision for much of their life.

The prevalence of USH varies from country to country and among ethnic groups, but is estimated to be about 4–5 individuals with USH per 100,000 births [9]. Types 1 and 2 account for the majority of USH in many countries, while only approximately 2% of all USH is type 3. The Finish population is an exception where USH3 accounts for about 40% of all USH cases [10]. A higher than expected frequency of a particular trait or disorder in a population is often due to a founder effect [11], which is discussed below as it relates to the genetics of USH.

Clinical Evaluation of Hearing in USH Patients

The onset, degree and progression of sensorineural hearing loss (SNHL) contribute to the clinical distinction between the three types of USH. Individuals with USH1 have congenital, severe-to-profound SNHL with residual hearing often limited to the low frequencies (fig. 1a) resulting in no useful hearing for speech recognition. Hearing loss in USH1 is stable, although there are reports of atypical cases with progressive hearing loss [12, 13]. USH2 is characterized by a congenital, down-sloping, moderate-to-severe SNHL (fig. 1a). While most reports describe stable hearing, several studies of cohorts with genetically confirmed USH2 have demonstrated progression of pure tone thresholds at a rate slightly greater than what can be accounted for by aging [14, 15]. In those with USH3, there is a progressive SNHL (fig. 1b) that is typically post lingual in onset, although the age of detection ranges from infancy to over 35 years with the majority identified by 10 years of age. In some cases, visual symptoms may precede the onset of hearing loss [16]. The audiometric configuration is most often down-sloping, and the degree of hearing loss can range from mild-to-moderate to profound [16, 17]. There is considerable heterogeneity in the degree and rate of hearing loss progression in USH3. Substantial progression may occur between the first and second decades, and again between the fourth and fifth decades [17], although this pattern is not universal.

The minimum test battery for hearing as recommended by the Usher Syndrome Consortium consists of tuning fork tests, determination of pure tone thresholds, white noise screening for islands of hearing, and speech discrimination measures. Comprehensive assessments includes tympanometry, measurement of the acoustic reflex, otoacoustic emissions, speech audiometry, auditory brainstem responses, electrocochleography, and cochlear implant assessment for implant candidates [7].

Because of the congenital onset of hearing loss, individuals with USH1 and USH2 will typically not pass a newborn hearing screening. Timely diagnostic testing is imperative to identify hearing loss sufficient to interfere with acquisition of speech and language skills and ensure early intervention for appropriate habilitation. Hearing aids may provide limited benefit and are often rejected by those with USH1, while those with USH2 and early USH3 frequently use hearing aids successfully. Cochlear implants have been used successfully in patients with all types of USH. Early cochlear implantation is important to maximize acquisition of speech and language skills and ensure central auditory development during critically sensitive periods in young children [18, 19].

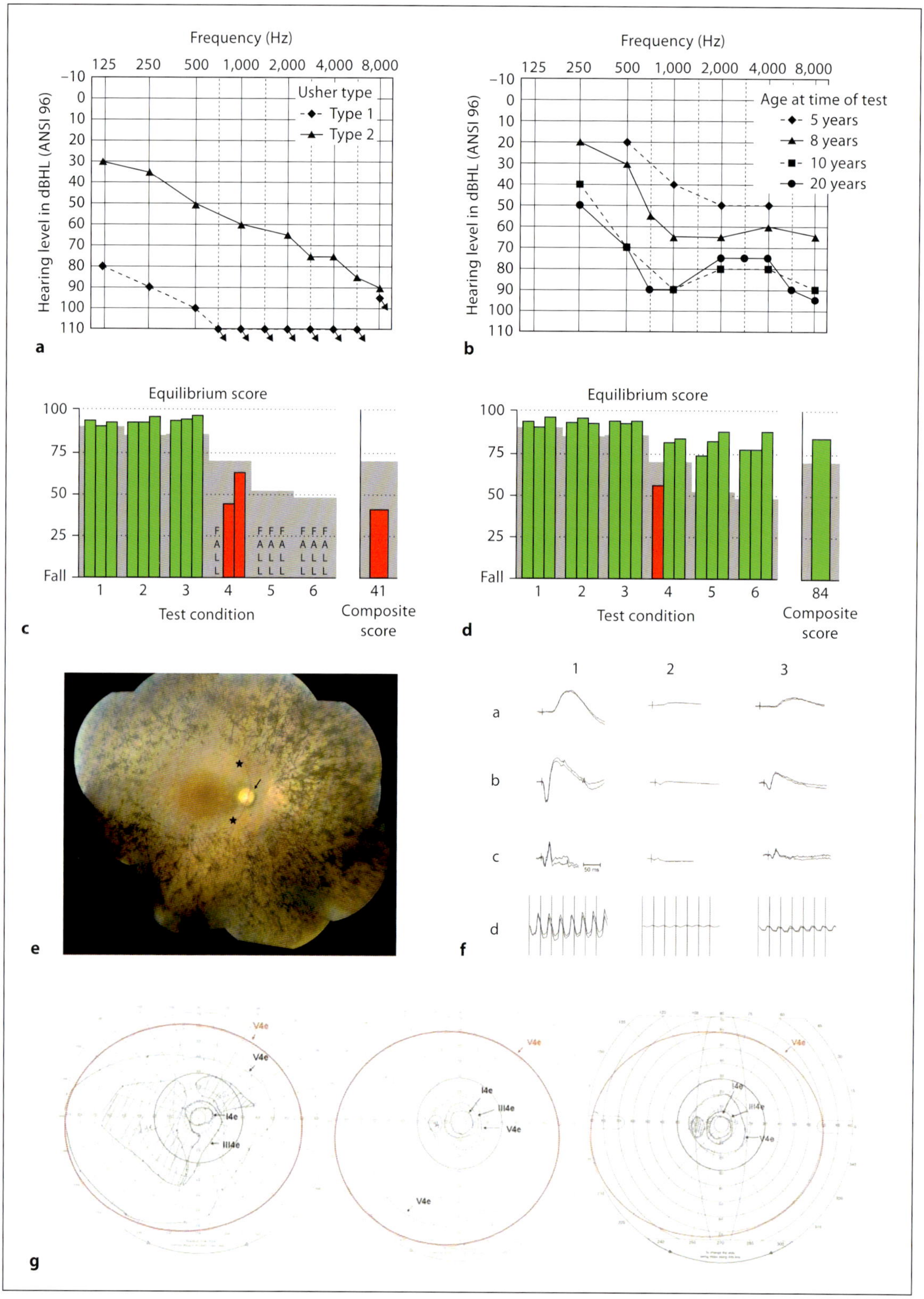
Frequency (Hz)
125 250 500 1,000 2,000 4,000 8,000
Hearing level in dBHL (ANSI 96)
–10 0 10 20 30 40 50 60 70 80 90 100 110
Usher type
Type 1
Type 2
a
Frequency (Hz)
125 250 500 1,000 2,000 4,000 8,000
Hearing level in dBHL (ANSI 96)
Age at time of test
5 years
8 years
10 years
20 years
b
Equilibrium score
100 75 50 25 Fall
1 2 3 4 5 6
Test condition
41
Composite score
c
Equilibrium score
100 75 50 25 Fall
1 2 3 4 5 6
Test condition
84
Composite score
d
e
1 2 3
a b c d
50 ms
f
V4e
I4e
III4e
g

This is an important consideration for those who will develop significant visual limitations later in life.

Clinical Evaluation of Vestibular Function in USH Patients

Individuals with USH1 have bilateral hypofunction or absence of a response to bithermal and ice water caloric stimulation of the horizontal semicircular canals [7, 20], and absent or reduced responses to sinusoidal harmonic acceleration on rotary chair testing [3]. Performance on the sensory organization test of computerized platform posturography results in falls when visual and somatosensory feedback is inaccurate and/or denied [3] (fig. 1c). This pattern is typical of those with bilaterally absent peripheral vestibular function. Late onset of independent walking and other delays in motor milestones are common in children with USH1 [3, 18]. The combination of motor delays and severe-to-profound congenital hearing loss should raise concern for possible Usher syndrome, especially in cases for whom structural abnormalities of the inner ear have been ruled out, for example enlarged vestibular aqueduct (EVA).

Vestibular function is normal in those with USH2 as evidenced by normal responses to caloric stimulation [7] and sinusoidal harmonic acceleration, normal function on oculomotor tests, and the absence of gaze and spontaneous nystagmus [3]. Performance on the sensory organization test of posturography is typically normal (fig. 1d). Results of vestibular assessments of individuals with USH3 indicate variable function. Caloric hypofunction or areflexia, reduced vestibulo-ocular response to sinusoidal harmonic acceleration, and/or abnormal performance on the sensory organization test of posturography occur in approximately 45% of those with USH3 [17]. Age of onset of independent walking is normal in most, although delays have been reported in a few with USH3 [17]. Longitudinal data tracking of vestibular function may provide additional insight into the onset and progression of vestibular dysfunction in this group.

The minimum test battery for vestibular evaluation should include Bruininks-Oseretsky tests of balance function including heel-toe walking, rail walking and rail standing; assessment of deep tendon reflexes, dysdiadochokinesia, and gait; and caloric stimulation with ice water. Comprehensive testing should include neuro-otologic evaluation, electro(video)nystagmography, rotary testing, and postural study [7]. Functional assessment of vestibular integrity in congenitally deaf children may provide an early opportunity to identify Usher syndrome. Screening procedures employing an abbreviated rotary chair test [21] or vestibular myogenic evoked potentials may become a routine part of the vestibular test battery.

Fig. 1. a, b Characteristic pure tone air-conduction thresholds. **a** USH1 (diamond) showing a severe to profound hearing loss with no response (arrow) at frequencies 1,000 Hz and above, and USH2 (triangle) showing a down-sloping hearing loss that ranges from mild in the low frequencies to severe in the high frequencies. **b** USH3 in which progressive hearing loss is documented over a 15 year time period. **c, d** Characteristic vestibular findings on Sensory Organization Test of Computerized Platform Posturography. Results are shown for each of three trials for six test conditions: (1) stable platform, eyes opened, (2) stable platform, eyes closed, (3) stable platform, moving visual surround, (4) moving platform, eyes opened, (5) moving platform, eyes closed, and (6) moving platform, moving visual surround, and as a composite score for USH1 (**c**) and USH2 (**d**). Equilibrium scores that are green are normal; those that are red are not normal; the gray shading represents the abnormal range. **e–g** Characteristic ocular findings in USH. **e** Fundoscopic findings: optic nerve pallor (arrow), vascular attenuation (stars), bone spicules and retinal pigment epithelial atrophy in the retinal periphery. **f** Full-field ERG responses (a) rod mediated, (b) rod and cone mediated (c), cone mediated, and (d) flicker from two USH1 patients (2 and 3) and a normal subject (1) for comparison. **g** Typical Goldmann kinetic visual fields in different stages of disease progression (red line represents a normal Goldmann visual field with V4e stimulus for comparison).

The complex interaction of the somatosensory, visual and vestibular systems in maintenance of balance is of concern in Usher syndrome in which one or two of these systems are compromised. The functional impact of vestibular dysfunction in USH1 and USH3 may be manifested as difficulty walking in the dark or on uneven surfaces, and clumsiness [3]. This becomes a greater problem as vision declines and raises concern for fall risk.

Clinical Evaluation of Retinal Function in USH Patients

RP is part of the clinical presentation of all three types of USH. The onset of ocular symptomatology is earlier in USH1 with patients perceiving night blindness in the first decade of life or the beginning of the second decade, while patients with USH2 usually report the beginning of symptoms towards the middle to end of the second decade. The time of initial presentation is more variable in patients with USH3. Despite the described differences, the time of onset of the visual symptoms cannot be considered a reliable diagnostic discriminator among the three types.

The initial visual symptom in all three types is usually difficulty with night vision that slowly expands to include constriction of visual fields, color vision defects and, in end-stage disease, decrease of visual acuity. Opinions differ as to whether the severity of the degeneration is different among the three clinical types [3, 22–24]. Detailed genotype-ophthalmic phenotype correlations exist for some USH alleles [25–29].

The minimum test battery as defined by the Usher Syndrome Consortium [7] consists of funduscopic examination, which reveals the characteristic findings of RP: optic nerve pallor, attenuated vessels, intraretinal pigment migration in the form of bone spicules or pigment clumps and retinal pigment epithelial atrophy (fig. 1e). Posterior subcapsular cataract, optic nerve drusen, atrophic foveal lesions, cellophane maculopathy, and cystoid macular edema are also often encountered. The prevalence of cystoid macular edema is higher if ocular cohererence tomography (OCT) or fluorescein angiography is employed [30].

In the absence of ophthalmoscopic findings but where there is a strong suspicion of USH, a comprehensive test battery is suggested, which includes visual field testing and electroretinography (ERG). Visual fields show variable degrees of constriction in different stages of the disease (fig. 1g). The final confirmation of the retinal degeneration is done with ERG, which for USH patients will show a decrease in the amplitude and delay in the implicit time of rod and cone responses (fig. 1f). ERG is the most sensitive test for the detection of the retinal degeneration and should always be done in the absence of the classic ophthalmoscopic findings, if USH is strongly suspected. ERG can be abnormal as early as infancy and before abnormalities are seen on fundoscopic examination [8, 18, 31].

Genetics of USH

Just as USH is clinically heterogeneous, it is also heterogeneous at the genetic level (table 1). Eleven loci for USH have been mapped and nine *USH* genes have been identified (table 1). There are many different recessive mutant alleles of some of these *USH* genes. A database has been established to keep track of all the published mutant alleles [32] (https://grenada.lumc.nl/LOVD2/Usher_montpellier/USHbases.html).

In the populations where USH has been studied, the majority of reported mutations are found in *MYO7A* (*USH1B*), *CDH23* (*USH1D*) and *USH2A* [32]. Most of these mutations are private, although there are common USH founder mutations segregating in some communities (table 2). For example, the p.Arg245X mutation of *PCDH15* and the p.Asn48Lys mutation of *USH3A* cause the majority of USH1 and USH3, respectively, in Ashkenazi Jews. Knowing the ethnicity of an USH patient has

Table 1. USH loci, genes, proteins and mouse models

Usher locus	OMIM[1]	Chromosome location	Gene	Protein	Non-syndromic deafness or RP[2]	Mouse model
USH1B	276900	11q13.5	*MYO7A*	myosin VIIA	*DFNB2, DFNA11*	shaker 1 (*sh1*)
USH1C	276904	11p15.1	*USH1C*	harmonin	*DFNB18*	deaf circler (*dfcr*)
USH1D	601067	10q22.1	*CDH23*	cadherin 23	*DFNB12*	waltzer (*v*)
USH1E	602097	21q21	not reported			
USH1F	602083	10q21.1	*PCDH15*	protocadherin 15	*DFNB23*	Ames waltzer (*av*)
USH1G	606943	17q25.1	*USH1G*	SANS		Jackson shaker (*js*)
USH1H	612632	15q22-q23	not reported			
USH2A	276901	1q41	*USH2A*	usherin	*RP39*	knockout
USH2C	605472	5q14.3	*GPR98*	G protein-coupled receptor 98		Frings, BUB/BnJ, Vlgr1/del7TM
USH2D	611383	9q32	*WHRN*	whirlin	*DFNB31*	Whirler (*wi*)
USH3A	276902	3q25.1	*CLRN1*	clarin-1		knockout

[1] Online Mendelian Inheritance in Man, http://www.ncbi.nlm.nih.gov/sites/entrez?db=omim.
[2] Particular mutations of genes associated with USH can also cause non-syndromic deafness or non-syndromic RP.

Table 2. Common and founder mutations associated with USH

Gene	Mutation	Population	Reference
USH1C	c.216G>A; p.Val72Val	Acadians and French Canadians from Quebec	[47]
CDH23	c.4504C>T; p.Arg1502X	Swedes	[12]
PCDH15	c.733C>T; p.Arg245X	Ashkenazi Jews	[1, 48]
USH2A	c.2299delG; p.Glu767fsX21	widespread	[49]
USH3A	c.143T>G; p.Asn48Lys	Ashkenazi Jews	[16, 50]
USH3A	c.528T>G; p.Tyr176X	Finns	[50]

practical value for genetic counselors and molecular geneticists.

The proteins encoded by the *USH* genes perform different functions and include unconventional myosin VIIa (USH1B), three scaffold proteins (harmonin, USH1C; whirlin, USH2D; SANS, USH1G), three adhesion proteins (cadherin 23, USH1D; protocadherin 15, USH1F; usherin, USH2A), the G protein-coupled receptor 98 (USH2C) and a synaptic protein (clarin-1, USH3A). In sensory cells of the retina and inner ear hair cells, many of the USH proteins interact with one another, partnering to form what has been called the Usher protein network [5]. For example, in hair cells, protocadherin 15 and cadherin 23 interaction is necessary for inner ear hair cell stereocilia bundle cohesion and tip link formation [33, 34]. Similarly, usherin and G protein-coupled receptor 98 constitute the transient ankle links which are located near the base of stereocilia. In the retina, myosin VIIa, harmonin, cadherin 23, protocadherin 15, and clarin-1 are localized at the ribbon synapses as well as in the connecting cilium of the photoreceptor cells. Recent studies show a common interacting partner, Nlp, for both usherin and lebercilin, a protein mutated in patients with Leber congenital amaurosis [35]. Based on these interactions and localization of USH proteins in the photoreceptor-connecting cilia, the RP component of USH may be thought of as a ciliopathy [35, 36].

Genotype-Phenotype Correlation for USH Genes

Genetic studies have provided insight into the clinical variation of USH. Some mutations of five of the six *USH1* genes do not result in RP but cause only non-syndromic deafness (table 1). In comparison to the retina, the auditory system seems to be more sensitive to small perturbations in the function of the USH proteins. For example, while all of the mutations of *CDH23* that truncate the protein cause USH1, some amino acid substitutions (missense mutations) of *CDH23* result only in deafness unaccompanied by RP and vestibular dysfunction, even late in life [12, 37]. Mutations of *USH* genes associated with non-syndromic deafness have also been reported for *MYO7A*, *USH1C*, *PCDH15*, and *WHRN* (table 1). Residual function of mutant myosin VIIA was found to be associated with non-syndromic deafness *DFNB2* [38].

The genetic background can also influence the phenotype. For example, in a family segregating a missense mutation of *CDH23* the hearing loss was variable. Affected individuals in this family also segregating a dominant modifier mutation in *PMCA2* encoding a plasma membrane calcium pump [39] have a more severe hearing loss. Thus, the severity of the hearing phenotype can be dependent on modifier genes.

Why Are There No USH1 Mouse Models?

Although in humans there is a genotype-phenotype relationship with less severe mutations associated with non-syndromic deafness; in mice, mutations of the orthologous human *USH1* genes cause only deafness (table 1), regardless of the mutation type. The *Ush2a* knockout mouse is the only model that mimics the phenotype seen in USH2A, exhibiting progressive photoreceptor degeneration and moderate, non-progressive, hearing impairment [40]. Some mouse models of other *USH* genes do very weakly recapitulate the human retinal degeneration. The retinas of six of nine *sh1* mutations of *Myo7a* that were examined by ERG showed a reduction of 20 to 30% in the a- and b-wave amplitudes [41]. Also, nine-month old *dfcr (Ush1c)* mutant mice have a mild peripheral photoreceptor degeneration, which is not accompanied by a reduction in ERG [42]. There is a reduction of ERG a- and b-wave amplitudes (~40%) at 5 weeks of age in at least two *(*$Pcdh15^{av\text{-}5J}$ and $Pcdh15^{av\text{-}jfb}$*)* of the seven *av* alleles with no RP [43]. A rodent model fully recapitulating the

RP component of USH1 will be valuable if not key to the development of somatic cell gene replacement in USH1 patients [44]. USH1 animal models will also be important to identify and study the safety and efficacy of therapeutic targets for small molecules [45, 46] that may prevent vision loss.

Acknowledgements

We thank Byung Yoon Choi, Penelope Friedman, Kelly King and Chris Zalewski for suggestions. This work was supported by the intramural program of the NIDCD/NIH projects Z01-DC00060–07 and Z01-DC00064–07 to Andrew J. Griffith, and Z01-DC000039–13 to T.B.F.

References

1 Brownstein Z, Ben-Yosef T, Dagan O, Frydman M, Abeliovich D, Sagi M, Abraham FA, Taitelbaum-Swead R, Shohat M, Hildesheimer M, Friedman TB, Avraham KB: The R245X mutation of PCDH15 in Ashkenazi Jewish children diagnosed with non-syndromic hearing loss foreshadows retinitis pigmentosa. Pediatr Res 2004;55:995–1000.

2 Ahmed ZM, Riazuddin S, Wilcox ER: The molecular genetics of Usher syndrome. Clin Genet 2003;63:431–444.

3 Moller CG, Kimberling WJ, Davenport SL, Priluck I, White V, Biscone-Halterman K, Odkvist LM, Brookhouser PE, Lund G, Grissom TJ: Usher syndrome: an otoneurologic study. Laryngoscope 1989;99:73–79.

4 Saihan Z, Webster AR, Luxon L, Bitner-Glindzicz M: Update on Usher syndrome. Curr Opin Neurol 2009;22: 19–27.

5 Adato A, Michel V, Kikkawa Y, Reiners J, Alagramam KN, Weil D, Yonekawa H, Wolfrum U, El-Amraoui A, Petit C: Interactions in the network of Usher syndrome type 1 proteins. Hum Mol Genet 2005;14:347–356.

6 Maerker T, van Wijk E, Overlack N, Kersten FF, McGee J, Goldmann T, Sehn E, Roepman R, Walsh EJ, Kremer H, Wolfrum U: A novel Usher protein network at the periciliary reloading point between molecular transport machineries in vertebrate photoreceptor cells. Hum Mol Genet 2008;17:71–86.

7 Smith RJ, Berlin CI, Hejtmancik JF, Keats BJ, Kimberling WJ, Lewis RA, Moller CG, Pelias MZ, Tranebjaerg L: Clinical diagnosis of the Usher syndromes. Usher Syndrome Consortium. Am J Med Genet 1994;50:32–38.

8 Young NM, Mets MB, Hain TC: Early diagnosis of Usher syndrome in infants and children. Am J Otol 1996;17:30–34.

9 Boughman JA, Vernon M, Shaver KA: Usher syndrome: definition and estimate of prevalence from two high-risk populations. J Chron Dis 1983;36:595–603.

10 Pakarinen L, Tuppurainen K, Laippala P, Mantyjarvi M, Puhakka H: The ophthalmological course of Usher syndrome type III. Int Ophthalmol 1995;19:307–311.

11 Drayna D: Founder mutations. Sci Am 2005;293:78–85.

12 Astuto LM, Bork JM, Weston MD, et al: CDH23 mutation and phenotype heterogeneity: a profile of 107 diverse families with Usher syndrome and nonsyndromic deafness. Am J Hum Genet 2002;71:262–275.

13 Liu XZ, Hope C, Walsh J, Newton V, Ke XM, Liang CY, Xu LR, Zhou JM, Trump D, Steel KP, Bundey S, Brown SD: Mutations in the myosin VIIA gene cause a wide phenotypic spectrum, including atypical Usher syndrome. Am J Hum Genet 1998;63:909–912.

14 Bernal S, Meda C, Solans T, Ayuso C, Garcia-Sandoval B, Valverde D, Del Rio E, Baiget M: Clinical and genetic studies in Spanish patients with Usher syndrome type II: description of new mutations and evidence for a lack of genotype-phenotype correlation. Clin Genet 2005;68:204–214.

15 Pennings RJ, Huygen PL, Weston MD, van Aarem A, Wagenaar M, Kimberling WJ, Cremers CW: Pure tone hearing thresholds and speech recognition scores in Dutch patients carrying mutations in the USH2A gene. Otol Neurotol 2003;24:58–63.

16 Ness SL, Ben-Yosef T, Bar-Lev A, Madeo AC, Brewer CC, Avraham KB, Kornreich R, Desnick RJ, Willner JP, Friedman TB, Griffith AJ: Genetic homogeneity and phenotypic variability among Ashkenazi Jews with Usher syndrome type III. J Med Genet 2003;40:767–772.

17 Sadeghi M, Cohn ES, Kimberling WJ, Tranebjaerg L, Moller C: Audiological and vestibular features in affected subjects with USH3: a genotype/phenotype correlation. Int J Audiol 2005;44:307–316.

18 Mets MB, Young NM, Pass A, Lasky JB: Early diagnosis of Usher syndrome in children. Trans Am Ophthalmol Soc 2000;98:237–242.

19 Sharma A, Dorman MF, Kral A: The influence of a sensitive period on central auditory development in children with unilateral and bilateral cochlear implants. Hear Res 2005;203:134–143.

20 Kumar A, Fishman G, Torok N: Vestibular and auditory function in Usher's syndrome. Ann Otol Rhinol Laryngol 1984;93:600–608.

21 Teschner M, Neuburger J, Gockeln R, Lenarz T, Lesinski-Schiedat A: 'Minimized rotational vestibular testing' as a screening procedure detecting vestibular areflexy in deaf children: screening cochlear implant candidates for Usher syndrome type I. Eur Arch Otorhinolaryngol 2008;265:759–763.

22 Sadeghi AM, Eriksson K, Kimberling WJ, Sjostrom A, Moller C: Longterm visual prognosis in Usher syndrome types 1 and 2. Acta Ophthalmol Scand 2006;84:537–544.

23 Seeliger M, Pfister M, Gendo K, Paasch S, Apfelstedt-Sylla E, Plinkert P, Zenner HP, Zrenner E: Comparative study of visual, auditory, and olfactory function in Usher syndrome. Graefes Arch Clin Exp Ophthalmol 1999;237:301–307.

24 Tsilou ET, Rubin BI, Caruso RC, Reed GF, Pikus A, Hejtmancik JF, Iwata F, Redman JB, Kaiser-Kupfer MI: Usher syndrome clinical types I and II: could ocular symptoms and signs differentiate between the two types? Acta Ophthalmol Scand 2002;80:196–201.

25 Herrera W, Aleman TS, Cideciyan AV, Roman AJ, Banin E, Ben-Yosef T, Gardner LM, Sumaroka A, Windsor EA, Schwartz SB, Stone EM, Liu XZ, Kimberling WJ, Jacobson SG: Retinal disease in Usher syndrome III caused by mutations in the clarin-1 gene. Invest Ophthalmol Vis Sci 2008;49:2651–2660.
26 Pennings RJ, Huygen PL, Orten DJ, Wagenaar M, van Aarem A, Kremer H, Kimberling WJ, Cremers CW, Deutman AF: Evaluation of visual impairment in Usher syndrome 1b and Usher syndrome 2a. Acta Ophthalmol Scand 2004;82: 131–139.
27 Plantinga RF, Pennings RJ, Huygen PL, Sankila EM, Tuppurainen K, Kleemola L, Cremers CW, Deutman AF: Visual impairment in Finnish Usher syndrome type III. Acta Ophthalmol Scand 2006; 84:36–41.
28 Sandberg MA, Rosner B, Weigel-DiFranco C, McGee TL, Dryja TP, Berson EL: Disease course in patients with autosomal recessive retinitis pigmentosa due to the USH2A gene. Invest Ophthalmol Vis Sci 2008;49:5532–5539.
29 Schwartz SB, Aleman TS, Cideciyan AV, Windsor EA, Sumaroka A, Roman AJ, Rane T, Smilko EE, Bennett J, Stone EM, Kimberling WJ, Liu XZ, Jacobson SG: Disease expression in Usher syndrome caused by VLGR1 gene mutation (USH2C) and comparison with USH2A phenotype. Invest Ophthalmol Vis Sci 2005;46:734–743.
30 Walia S, Fishman GA, Hajali M: Prevalence of cystic macular lesions in patients with Usher II syndrome. Eye (Lond) 2009;23:1206–1209.
31 Flores-Guevara R, Renault F, Loundon N, Marlin S, Pelosse B, Momtchilova M, Auzoux-Cheve M, Vermersch AI, Richard P: Usher syndrome type 1: early detection of electroretinographic changes. Eur J Paediatr Neurol 2009;13: 505–507.
32 Baux D, Faugere V, Larrieu L, Le Guedard-Mereuze S, Hamroun D, Beroud C, Malcolm S, Claustres M, Roux AF: UMD-USHbases: a comprehensive set of databases to record and analyse pathogenic mutations and unclassified variants in seven Usher syndrome causing genes. Hum Mutat 2008;29:E76–E87.
33 Ahmed ZM, Goodyear R, Riazuddin S, Lagziel A, Legan PK, Behra M, Burgess SM, Lilley KS, Wilcox ER, Griffith AJ, Frolenkov GI, Belyantseva IA, Richardson GP, Friedman TB: The tip-link antigen, a protein associated with the transduction complex of sensory hair cells, is protocadherin-15. J Neurosci 2006;26:7022–7034.
34 Kazmierczak P, Sakaguchi H, Tokita J, Wilson-Kubalek EM, Milligan RA, Muller U, Kachar B: Cadherin 23 and protocadherin 15 interact to form tip-link filaments in sensory hair cells. Nature 2007;449:87–91.
35 van Wijk E, Kersten FF, Kartono A, Mans DA, Brandwijk K, Letteboer SJ, Peters TA, Marker T, Yan X, Cremers CW, Cremers FP, Wolfrum U, Roepman R, Kremer H: Usher syndrome and Leber congenital amaurosis are molecularly linked via a novel isoform of the centrosomal ninein-like protein. Hum Mol Genet 2009;18:51–64.
36 Williams DS: Usher syndrome: animal models, retinal function of Usher proteins, and prospects for gene therapy. Vision Res 2008;48:433–441.
37 Bork JM, Peters LM, Riazuddin S, et al: Usher syndrome 1D and non-syndromic autosomal recessive deafness DFNB12 are caused by allelic mutations of the novel cadherin-like gene CDH23. Am J Hum Genet 2001;68:26–37.
38 Riazuddin S, Nazli S, Ahmed ZM, Yang Y, Zulfiqar F, Shaikh RS, Zafar AU, Khan SN, Sabar F, Javid FT, Wilcox ER, Tsilou E, Boger ET, Sellers JR, Belyantseva IA, Friedman TB: Mutation spectrum of MYO7A and evaluation of a novel nonsyndromic deafness DFNB2 allele with residual function. Hum Mutat 2008;29: 502–511.
39 Schultz JM, Yang Y, Caride AJ, Filoteo AG, Penheiter AR, Lagziel A, Morell RJ, Mohiddin SA, Fananapazir L, Madeo AC, Penniston JT, Griffith AJ: Modification of human hearing loss by plasma-membrane calcium pump PMCA2. N Engl J Med 2005;352:1557–1564.
40 Liu X, Bulgakov OV, Darrow KN, Pawlyk B, Adamian M, Liberman MC, Li T: Usherin is required for maintenance of retinal photoreceptors and normal development of cochlear hair cells. Proc Natl Acad Sci USA 2007;104:4413–4418.
41 Gibbs D, Kitamoto J, Williams DS: Abnormal phagocytosis by retinal pigmented epithelium that lacks myosin VIIa, the Usher syndrome 1B protein. Proc Natl Acad Sci USA 2003;100:6481–6486.
42 Johnson KR, Gagnon LH, Webb LS, Peters LL, Hawes NL, Chang B, Zheng QY: Mouse models of USH1C and DFNB18: phenotypic and molecular analyses of two new spontaneous mutations of the Ush1c gene. Hum Mol Genet 2003;12:3075–3086.
43 Haywood-Watson RJ 2nd, Ahmed ZM, Kjellstrom S, Bush RA, Takada Y, Hampton LL, Battey JF, Sieving PA, Friedman TB: Ames Waltzer deaf mice have reduced electroretinogram amplitudes and complex alternative splicing of Pcdh15 transcripts. Invest Ophthalmol Vis Sci 2006;47:3074–3084.
44 Jacobson SG, Cideciyan AV, Aleman TS, Sumaroka A, Roman AJ, Gardner LM, Prosser HM, Mishra M, Bech-Hansen NT, Herrera W, Schwartz SB, Liu XZ, Kimberling WJ, Steel KP, Williams DS: Usher syndromes due to MYO7A, PCDH15, USH2A or GPR98 mutations share retinal disease mechanism. Hum Mol Genet 2008;17:2405–2415.
45 Nudelman I, Rebibo-Sabbah A, Cherniavsky M, Belakhov V, Hainrichson M, Chen F, Schacht J, Pilch DS, Ben-Yosef T, Baasov T: Development of novel aminoglycoside (NB54) with reduced toxicity and enhanced suppression of disease-causing premature stop mutations. J Med Chem 2009;52:2836–2845.
46 Rebibo-Sabbah A, Nudelman I, Ahmed ZM, Baasov T, Ben-Yosef T: In vitro and ex vivo suppression by aminoglycosides of PCDH15 nonsense mutations underlying type 1 Usher syndrome. Hum Genet 2007;122:373–381.
47 Ebermann I, Lopez I, Bitner-Glindzicz M, Brown C, Koenekoop RK, Bolz HJ: Deafblindness in French Canadians from Quebec: a predominant founder mutation in the USH1C gene provides the first genetic link with the Acadian population. Genome Biol 2007;8:R47.

48 Ben-Yosef T, Ness SL, Madeo AC, Bar-Lev A, Wolfman JH, Ahmed ZM, Desnick RJ, Willner JP, Avraham KB, Ostrer H, Oddoux C, Griffith AJ, Friedman TB: A mutation of PCDH15 among Ashkenazi Jews with the type 1 Usher syndrome. N Engl J Med 2003; 348:1664–1670.

49 Dreyer B, Tranebjaerg L, Brox V, Rosenberg T, Moller C, Beneyto M, Weston MD, Kimberling WJ, Cremers CW, Liu XZ, Nilssen O: A common ancestral origin of the frequent and widespread 2299delG USH2A mutation. Am J Hum Genet 2001;69:228–234.

50 Fields RR, Zhou G, Huang D, Davis JR, Moller C, Jacobson SG, Kimberling WJ, Sumegi J: Usher syndrome type III: revised genomic structure of the USH3 gene and identification of novel mutations. Am J Hum Genet 2002;71:607–617.

Thomas B. Friedman, PhD
5 Research Court, Rm 2A-19, NIDCD, NIH
Rockville, MD 20850 (USA)
Tel. +1 301 496 7882, Fax +1 301 402 7580, E-Mail friedman@nidcd.nih.gov

Alford RL, Sutton VR (eds): Medical Genetics in the Clinical Practice of ORL.
Adv Otorhinolaryngol. Basel, Karger, 2011, vol 70, pp 66–74

Genetic Disorders with both Hearing Loss and Cardiovascular Abnormalities

John W. Belmont · William J. Craigen · Hugo Martinez · John Lynn Jefferies

Departments of Molecular and Human Genetics, and Pediatrics, Baylor College of Medicine, Houston, Tex., USA

Abstract

There has been a growing appreciation for conditions that affect hearing and which are accompanied by significant cardiovascular disorders. In this chapter we consider several broad classes of conditions including deafness due to abnormal structural development of the inner ear, those with physiological abnormalities in the inner ear sensory apparatus, and conditions with progressive loss of function of sensory cells or middle ear functions. Because of shared developmental controls, inner ear malformations are often associated with congenital heart defects and can be part of complex syndromes that affect other organs and neurodevelopmental outcome. Physiological disorders of the hair cells can lead to hearing loss and can be associated with cardiac arrhythmias, especially long QT syndrome. In addition, cellular energy defects such as mitochondrial disorders can affect maintenance of hair cells and are often associated with cardiomyopathy. Lysosomal storage diseases and other disorders affecting connective tissue can lead to chronic middle ear disease, with conductive hearing loss and also cause cardiac valve disease and/or cardiomyopathy. The genetic basis for these conditions is heterogeneous and includes chromosomal/genomic disorders, de novo dominant mutations, and familial dominant, autosomal-recessive, and mitochondrial (matrilineal) inheritance. Taken together, there are more than 100 individual genes implicated in genetic hearing impairment that are also associated with congenital and/or progressive cardiac abnormalities. These genes encode transcription factors, chromatin remodeling factors, components of signal transduction pathways, ion channels, mitochondrial proteins and assembly factors, extracellular matrix proteins, and enzymes involved in lysosomal functions.

Defects of the Inner Ear Associated with Cardiovascular Malformations

Genomic Disorders

DiGeorge Syndrome and 22q11 Deletion. Occurring at a frequency of 1 in 4,000 live births, submicroscopic deletion of 22q11.2 occurs in approximately 90% of patients with DiGeorge syndrome [1]. Moreover, 22q11 deletion accounts for a spectrum of clinical conditions including Sprintzen syndrome, velocardiofacial syndrome, and rarely CHARGE, Opitz BBB, and oculoauriculovertebral syndromes. A significant number of common otolaryngologic problems are found in these syndromes. These include velopharyngeal insufficiency, cleft palate, characteristic facial dysmorphisms, otitis media, sinorhinitis, hearing loss, and speech and language difficulties [2, 3]. Cardiac malformations in 22q11 deletion syndrome are usually 'conotruncal', reflecting a consistent impact on the development of the common outflow tract of the embryonic heart. The resulting malformations can include tetralogy of Fallot (fig. 1a),

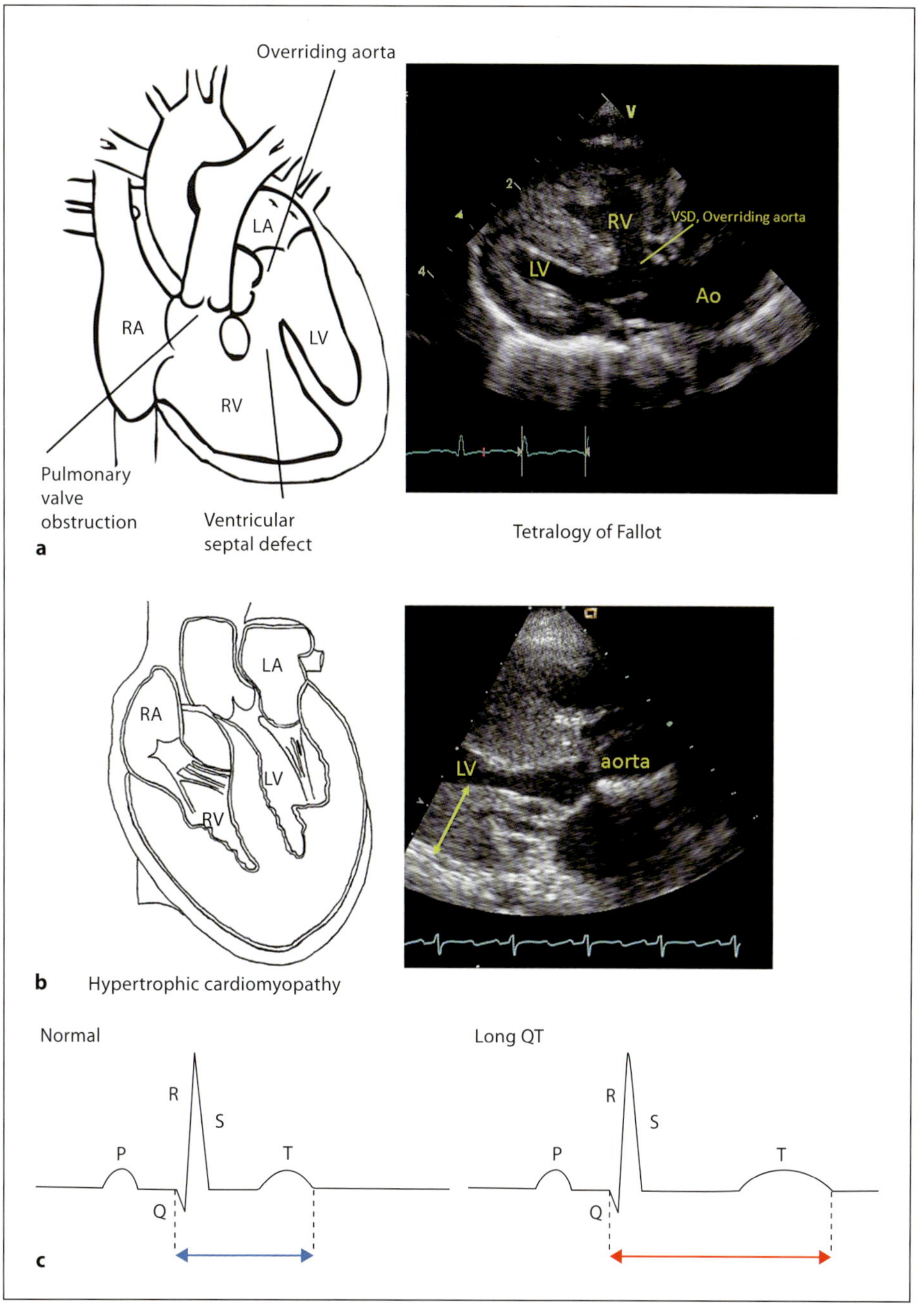

Fig. 1. a Tetralogy of Fallot – a typical conontruncal heart defect. Ventricular septal defect, overriding aorta, obstruction of the right outflow tract and right ventricular hypertrophy are the characteristic features of the lesion. **b** Hypertrophic cardiomyopathy is seen in the Noonan syndrome spectrum disorders and various metabolic or mitochondrial conditions. Note the extreme thickening of the ventricular myocardium. **c** Long QT syndromes have specific changes on EKG that include delayed and prolonged repolarization as indicated by the abnormal T wave.

interrupted aortic arch type B, double outlet right ventricle, perimembranous ventricular septal defects, and related anomalies [4]. Approximately 70% of children with 22q11 deletion have an associated heart defect.

1p36 Deletion Syndrome. Monosomy 1p36 is the most common terminal deletion syndrome, and is characterized by short stature, microcephaly, sensorineural deafness, renal abnormalities, seizures, developmental delay, and hypotonia. This disorder has a prevalence of 1 in 5,000 newborns and accounts for 0.5–1.2% of syndromic mental retardation [5]. Deafness is a characteristic finding in 1p36 deletion syndrome. In one study involving 52 patients, 77% showed hearing deficits, either conductive, sensorineural, or both [6]. Heart defects typically include dilated cardiomyopathy, left ventricular noncompaction, or ventricular septal defects. In a summary of published cases structural cardiac defects were noted in 73% and cardiomyopathy in 29% of 1p36 deletion syndrome patients [7]. The mechanisms that account for either the functional or structural cardiac disease remain to be established.

4p16 Deletion Syndrome. Wolf Hirschhorn syndrome (WHS) is caused by deletion of 4p16.3 [8]. It has a frequency of about 1/50,000 live births, with a female:male ratio of 2:1. The disorder is defined by characteristic dysmorphic facial features: prominent glabella, hypertelorism, beaked nose often described as 'Greek helmet' facies. Poor growth, cleft lip and palate, midline CNS defects, heart defects and genitourinary abnormalities are also common. No intragenic mutations have been shown to confer the full WHS phenotype. Ear anomalies are common in WHS, consisting of simple, posteriorly rotated and low-set ears, occasionally with lobeless pinnae or with underdeveloped/absent cartilage, or preauricular pits and tags. Some individuals have microtia. In one of the largest studies of the condition hearing loss was detected in just over 40% of the patients; conductive in 25%; and sensorineural in 15% [9]. One of the known genes for autosomal-dominant nonsyndromic hearing loss, *DFNA6*, [10] encoding the wolframin protein, maps to chromosome 4p16.3 in a region that is partially deleted in patients with WHS. The same gene, when biallelically mutated, causes one form of autosomal-recessive Wolfram syndrome, characterized by optic atrophy, deafness, diabetes insipidus, and occasionally cardiovascular malformations. Cardiac defects are also common in WHS, but there is not a characteristic lesion described [11].

6p24 Deletion Syndrome. Deletions involving terminal 6p are relatively rare with only about 30 cases described in the literature [12]. Features associated with the terminal deletions include anterior eye-chamber abnormalities, hypertelorism, mid-face hypoplasia, low-set ears, hearing loss, heart defects, and developmental delay. Deafness or auditory hypersensitivity has been observed in several patients [13]. Heart defects include aortic valve abnormalities, which may be attributed to deletion of the transcription factor FOXC1 as aortic valve abnormalities have been observed in Foxc1 mutant mice.

Williams Syndrome (Deletion 7q11.23). Williams syndrome (WS) has an estimated prevalence of 1 in 7,500–20,000 live births [14]. It is characterized by 'elfin' facial appearance, an unusually cheerful personality, cardiovascular abnormalities, growth deficiency, mild-to-moderate mental retardation and hypercalcemia [15]. Due to disruptions in the middle-ear system in this pathology, otitis media and the conductive hearing loss that frequently accompanies it may persist until adulthood [16]. High-frequency sensorineural hearing loss or mixed hearing in the mild to moderate range has been reported in about 60–70% in school-aged children with WS [17]. Supravalvar aortic stenosis (SVAS) and branch peripheral pulmonary arterial stenosis (PPS) are the most common cardiovascular abnormalities reported [18]. WS is caused by a hemizygous 1.5-Mb deletion including approximately 28 genes on chromosome 7q11.23 [18]. The deleted region at the *ELN* locus (which encodes elastin) on chromosome 7q11.23

has been demonstrated to be the cause of the vascular lesions in WS and in the nonsyndromic supravalvular aortic stenosis (SVAS) [18]. *ELN* has also been implicated in the impaired cochlear function [19].

Single Gene Disorders

CHARGE Syndrome. Pagon et al. [20] coined the acronym and summarized the six cardinal clinical features: ocular coloboma, heart defects of any type, atresia of the choanae, retardation (of growth and/or of development), genital anomalies and ear anomalies (abnormal pinnae or hearing loss). The incidence of CHARGE is about 1/8,500–12,500 [21]. All three segments of the ear are affected. In 95–100%, the pinnae are asymmetrically misshaped, low set, anteverted, cup-shaped, wide, but with reduced vertical height. Lack of cartilage produces short cup-shaped ears with hypoplastic lobules. Facial nerve palsies are also very common and correlated with sensorineural hearting loss. Absence of the stapedius muscle, absence of the oval window, and hypoplastic incus and stapes with ossicular chain fixation have been observed. More than 90% of CHARGE patients have a characteristic inner ear malformation called Mondini dysplasia [22, 23]. This consists of complete absence of the pars superior (utricle and semicircular canals) with or without involvement of the pars inferior (cochlea and saccule). Aplasia of the semicircular canals and hypoplastic uncus are probably the most specific anomalies of CHARGE syndrome. While these abnormalities may be observed as isolated defects, CHD7 sequencing should be considered in individuals these inner ear malformations. Deafness affects 60–90% of cases and is characterized by severe conductive or mixed loss [24]. Congenital heart defects occur in 75–80% of patients with CHARGE syndrome [25]. The most common major heart defect is tetralogy of Fallot (33%). Other frequent anomalies are double outlet right ventricle with atrioventricular canal, ventricular septal defect and atrial septal defect with or without cleft mitral valve. The chromodomain helicase DNA-binding protein 7 (*CHD7*) gene is mutated in about 60% of CHARGE cases [25]. More than 98% of mutations occur as de novo dominant mutations and most mutations are either nonsense or frameshift [26].

Townes-Brocks Syndrome. Townes-Brocks syndrome (TBS) is characterized by the triad of imperforate anus, triphalangeal and supernumerary thumbs, and ear malformations with deafness. However, the phenotype is variable, and TBS also has features that overlap with oculoauriculovertebral spectrum and VATER syndrome [27, 28]. Most TBS patients have deformities of the outer ear ('lop ears', microtia), preauricular tags, and hearing loss, which can be sensorineural, conductive, or mixed. Cardiac anomalies have been reported in 14% of cases (2% of familial cases, 10% probands, and 59% of sporadic cases). Major heart defects include truncus arteriosus, tetrology of Fallot, and atrial or ventricular septal defect. Sporadic cases show a higher percentage of cardiac anomalies and nervous system manifestations when compared to rare families affected with the condition. TBS was found to be caused by mutations within the *SALL1* transcription factor gene at 16q12.1 [29].

Axenfeld-Rieger Syndrome Type 3. Axenfeld-Rieger (AR) syndrome is an autosomal-dominant disorder of morphogenesis that results in abnormal development of the anterior segment of the eye and other anomalies including deafness (AR Type 3), dental abnormalities, and cardiovascular defects. The typical features of AR type 3 include flat midface, sensorineural hearing loss, iris hypoplasia, glaucoma, hypertelorism, and hypodontia. Cardiac abnormalities can include patent ductus arteriosus, atrial septal defect, and valvular defects. AR type 3 is caused by mutations in the *FOXC1* gene [30].

Noonan Syndrome. Noonan syndrome (NS) is a common autosomal-dominant disorder with an aggregate incidence of about 1 in 2,500 live births [31]. It is characterized by short stature, webbed neck, facial dysmorphism, learning disabilities, hearing loss, undescended testes and pubertal delay, variable coagulation defects, and heart defects. There is clinical overlap with cardio-facio-cutaneous, Costello and Leopard syndromes, and thus this group of conditions is often referred to as Noonan spectrum disorders [32]. See also the chapter by Toriello [this vol.]. Sensorineural hearing loss occurs in up to 25% of patients [33]. The most common congenital heart defect in NS is pulmonary valve stenosis with dysplastic leaflets (50–62%) [34]. Hypertrophic cardiomyopathy (HCM; fig. 1b) with asymmetric septum hypertrophy is present in 20% of patients. Other congenital heart defects more often seen in NS are atrioventricular canal defect) associated with subaortic obstruction and structural anomalies of the mitral valve. The genes that cause NS encode proteins of the Ras/MAPK signal transduction pathway that regulates cellular proliferation and differentiation [35]. Mutations in *PTPN11* are detected in 50% of individuals with NS. Mutations in the genes *RAF1, SOS1, KRAS, MAP2K1, MAP2K2, HRAS, NRAS, SHOC2, and BRAF* have also been reported in individuals with NS and the related disorders. No mutation is identified in 25–30% of NS patients, indicating still greater locus heterogeneity.

Sensorineural Hearing Loss with Cardiac Arrhythmia or Cardiomyopathy

Jervell-Lange Neilsen Syndrome. Long QT syndromes (LQTS) are genetic conditions characterized by prolonged QT intervals detected by electrocardiography and indicating delayed cardiac repolarization (fig. 1c). Jervell-Lange Nielsen syndrome (JLNS) is an uncommon autosomal-recessive subtype of LQTS (estimated prevalence 1:50,000) associated with congenital deafness. Sensorineural deafness is a uniform feature of JLNS. Marked atrophy of the stria vascularis and collapse of the endolymphatic compartments and surrounding membranes is observed the mouse model of *Kcnq1* mutation. There is also complete degeneration of the organ of Corti and associated degeneration of the spiral ganglion. A large cooperative study providing detailed clinical information on 187 JLNS patients has allowed the recognition of clear electrophysiologic differences in comparison to the other types of LQTS, including LQT1 [36]. JLNS is among the most severe of the major variants of LQTS. Approximately 90% of affected individuals have clinically significant arrhythmias, usually presenting by age 3 years. JLNS is a recessive disorder resulting from mutations in either the *KCNQ1* or *KCNE1* genes. The smaller group of patients with *KCNE1* mutations has a markedly less severe clinical course than those with mutations of *KCNQ1* [37]. An unusual feature of JLNS is that although the carriers are not affected with deafness they may be affected with LQTS.

Leopard Syndrome. Leopard syndrome (OMIM# 151100) is an autosomal-dominant disorder whose clinical features include multiple lentigines, electrocardiographic conduction abnormalities, ocular hypertelorism, pulmonic stenosis, abnormal genitalia, retardation of growth, and sensorineural deafness. There is clinical overlap with features of Noonan syndrome. Sensorineural deafness occurs in about 15–25% of patients. Most cases are diagnosed at birth or during childhood, but deafness may develop later in life [38]. About 70% of LS individuals display cardiac defects [39]. Hypertrophic cardiomyopathy (HCM) is the most frequent anomaly; detected in up to 80% of the patients with a cardiac defect [40]. Mutations in exons 7, 12 and 13 of *PTPN11* have been detected in the majority of individuals with Leopard syndrome (90–100%) [41, 42]. About 33% of patients who lack a *PTPN11* mutation have a mutation in either *RAF1* or *BRAF* [43, 44]. For further discussion of the dermatologic phenotype in Leopardsyndrome, see also the chapter by Toriello [this vol.].

Alstrom Syndrome. This disorder is characterized by progressive blindness (cone-rod dystrophy), sensorineural hearing loss, childhood obesity, and type 2 diabetes mellitus with insulin resistance [45]. The sensorineural hearing loss is evident in 70% within the first 10 years of life and is progressive. The hearing loss may progress to the severe or moderately severe range (40–70 db) by adulthood with 88% of individuals affected. Dilated cardiomyopathy occurs in 70% of patients and is progressive. Renal failure develops with age. The condition exhibits autosomal-recessive inheritance resulting from mutations in the *ALMS1* gene [46].

Refsum Disease. Refsum disease is an inborn error of metabolism leading to the accumulation of a very long chain fatty acid, phytanic acid, that causes retinitis pigmentosa, peripheral neuropathy, cerebellar ataxia, deafness and cardiomyopathy [47]. It can be diagnosed by measuring plasma phytanic acid levels.

Mitochondrial Disorders. Mitochondrial disorders are multi-organ diseases with a wide spectrum of clinical features and, because of the high energy requirements of the auditory and cardiovascular systems, often include deafness and cardiomyopathy. There are several well-described clinical syndromes that exemplify the intersection of otological and cardiac dysfunction in mitochondrial disorders.

MELAS – mitochondrial encephalopathy, lactic acidosis, and stroke-like episodes – primarily caused by a mtDNA-encoded tRNA mutation, may also be complicated by diabetes, epilepsy, dementia, ataxia, cortical blindness, optic atrophy, deafness, migraine, cardiac conduction defects (Wolf-Parkinson White syndrome) and cardiomyopathy [48].

MERRF – myoclonic epilepsy and ragged red fibers – caused by a different mtDNA-encoded tRNA mutation, typically presents with skeletal myopathy, ataxia, dementia, extra-ocular muscle disturbance called chronic progressive external ophthalmoplegia, deafness, epilepsy and dilated cardiomyopathy [49].

Wolfram syndrome (DIDMOAD) – diabetes insipidus, diabetes mellitus, optic atrophy, deafness, neurogenic bladder, intestinal dysmotility, may be due to mutations in the *WFS1* gene or the *CISD1* gene. *WFS1*-related sensorineural hearing loss is slowly progressive and particularly affects low-frequency (<2,000 Hz) hearing. Cisd1 functions as an iron binding protein to regulate the activity of the respiratory chain complex I NADH dehydrogenase [50]. *WFS1* encodes a protein that localizes to endoplasmic reticulum. This localization suggests physiological functions in membrane trafficking, secretion, processing and/or regulation of ER calcium homeostasis [51].

Kearns-Sayre syndrome – presents with ophthalmoplegia, degenerative retinopathy, renal tubular dysfunction, delayed growth, short stature, slow mental and neurologic deterioration, skeletal myopathy and progressive heart block. Less common features include deafness, bulbar symptoms, stroke-like episodes, endocrine dysfunction, and sideroblastic anaemia [52]. KSS is due to large deletions ranging from 1.3 to 8.8 kb (90% of the cases) or duplications in the mtDNA. It is typically a sporadic condition, although rare familial cases are described.

Mitochondrial complex I deficiency – reduced nicotinamide-adenine dinucleotide-coenzyme Q (NADH-CoQ) – causes three major clinical syndromes: fatal infantile multisystem disorder, myopathy, and mitochondrial encephalomyopathy. Cardiomyopathy has been observed clinically in infants with the fatal form in association with severe lactic acidosis, psychomotor delay, generalized hypotonia, and weakness. Deafness is a commonly observed complication in infants surviving the initial presentation of severe lactic acidemia [53]. Cardiac failure is the most common cause of death [54].

Conductive Hearing Loss with Cardiomyopathy or Cardiac Valve Disease

Mucopolysaccharidoses. Mucopolysaccharidoses are characterized by deficiencies in lysosomal enzymes involved in the degradation of various glycosaminoglycans. Because of progressive deposition of mucopolysaccharides, hearing loss, both conductive and sensorineural, is a very common finding in the mucopolysaccharidoses. Otological problems in mucopolysaccharidoses are complex, but most often include chronic middle ear infection/effusion and conductive hearing loss [55]. Cardiovascular lesions involve the valves, endocardium, myocardium, coronary arteries and large systemic arteries. The aortic and mitral valves are thickened and appose poorly leading to insufficiency [56]. Other lysosomal storage disorders such as sialidase deficiency, galactosialidosis, I cell disease, and mannosidosis can be similarly affected with both hearing loss and cardiovascular disease, including cardiomyopathy.

Osteogenesis Imperfecta. Osteogenesis imperfecta is a connective tissue disorder caused by defective synthesis of type I collagen. Clinical features include the blue sclera, pathologic fractures, conductive and sensorineural hearing loss, and dental abnormalities. Cardiovascular involvement is a less common feature but when present includes pathology of left-sided cardiac valves, the aortic root and ascending aorta. The most commonly reported cardiovascular abnormality is aortic root dilation with a prevalence of 12% [57].

References

1 Emanuel BS, McDonald-McGinn D, Saitta SC, Zackai EH: The 22q11.2 deletion syndrome. Adv Pediatr 2001;48: 39–73.
2 Vantrappen G, Rommel N, Swillen A, Cremers CW, Fryns JP, Devriendt K: Velo-cardio-facial syndrome: guidelines for diagnosis, treatment and follow-up of ent manifestations. Acta Otorhinolaryngol Belg 2003;57:101–106.
3 Dyce O, McDonald-McGinn D, Kirschner RE, Zackai E, Young K, Jacobs IN: Otolaryngologic manifestations of the 22q11.2 deletion syndrome. Arch Otolaryngol Head Neck Surg 2002;128: 1408–1412.
4 Momma K: Cardiovascular anomalies associated with chromosome 22q11.2 deletion syndrome. Am J Cardiol 2010;105:1617–1624.
5 Gajecka M, Mackay KL, Shaffer LG: Monosomy 1p36 deletion syndrome. Am J Med Genet C Semin Med Genet 2007; 145C:346–356.
6 Battaglia A, Hoyme HE, Dallapiccola B, Zackai E, Hudgins L, McDonald-McGinn D, Bahi-Buisson N, Romano C, Williams CA, Brailey LL, Zuberi SM, Carey JC: Further delineation of deletion 1p36 syndrome in 60 patients: a recognizable phenotype and common cause of developmental delay and mental retardation. Pediatrics 2008;121:404–410.
7 Rosenfeld JA, Crolla JA, Tomkins S, Bader P, Morrow B, Gorski J, Troxell R, Forster-Gibson C, Cilliers D, Hislop RG, Lamb A, Torchia B, Ballif BC, Shaffer LG: Refinement of causative genes in monosomy 1p36 through clinical and molecular cytogenetic characterization of small interstitial deletions. Am J Med Genet A 2010;152A:1951–1959.
8 Bergemann AD, Cole F, Hirschhorn K: The etiology of Wolf-Hirschhorn syndrome. Trends Genet 2005;21:188–195.
9 Ulualp SO, Wright CG, Pawlowski KS, Roland PS: Histopathological basis of hearing impairment in Wolf-Hirschhorn syndrome. Laryngoscope 2004;114: 1426–1430.
10 Lesperance MM, Grundfast KM, Rosenbaum KN: Otologic manifestations of Wolf-Hirschhorn syndrome. Arch Otolaryngol Head Neck Surg 1998;124: 193–196.
11 Battaglia A, Filippi T, Carey JC: Update on the clinical features and natural history of Wolf-Hirschhorn (4p-) syndrome: experience with 87 patients and recommendations for routine health supervision. Am J Med Genet C Semin Med Genet 2008;148C:246–251.
12 Lin RJ, Cherry AM, Chen KC, Lyons M, Hoyme HE, Hudgins L: Terminal deletion of 6p results in a recognizable phenotype. Am J Med Genet A 2005;136: 162–168.
13 Davies AF, Mirza G, Sekhon G, Turnpenny P, Leroy F, Speleman F, Law C, van Regemorter N, Vamos E, Flinter F, Ragoussis J: Delineation of two distinct 6p deletion syndromes. Hum Genet 1999;104:64–72.
14 Martens MA, Wilson SJ, Reutens DC: Research Review: Williams syndrome: a critical review of the cognitive, behavioral, and neuroanatomical phenotype. J Child Psychol Psychiatry 2008;49: 576–608.
15 Marler JA, Sitcovsky JL, Mervis CB, Kistler DJ, Wightman FL: Auditory function, hearing loss in children and adults with Williams syndrome: cochlear impairment in individuals with otherwise normal hearing. Am J Med Genet C 2010;154C:249–265.
16 Cherniske EM, Carpenter TO, Klaiman C, Young E, Bregman J, Insogna K, Schultz RT, Pober BR: Multisystem study of 20 older adults with Williams syndrome. Am J Med Genet A 2004;131: 255–264.
17 Marler JA, Elfenbein JL, Ryals BM, Urban Z, Netzloff ML: Sensorineural hearing loss in children and adults with Williams syndrome. Am J Med Genet A 2005;138:318–327.
18 Collins RT, 2nd, Kaplan P, Somes GW, Rome JJ: Cardiovascular abnormalities, interventions, and long-term outcomes in infantile Williams syndrome. J Pediatr 2010;156:253–258, e251.
19 Mikuni H, Ushiki T, Abe K, Fukuda S, Inuyama Y: Nature of the fine fibrils of the basilar membrane in the cochlea. Arch Histol Cytol 1994;57:187–191.

20 Pagon RA, Zonana J, Graham JM: CHARGE association. Pediatrics 1982; 70:827–828.
21 Sanlaville D, Verloes A: CHARGE syndrome: an update. Eur J Hum Genet 2007;15:389–399.
22 Wiener-Vacher SR, Amanou L, Denise P, Narcy P, Manach Y: Vestibular function in children with the CHARGE association. Arch Otolaryngol Head Neck Surg 1999;125:342–347.
23 Guyot JP, Gacek RR, DiRaddo P: The temporal bone anomaly in CHARGE association. Arch Otolaryngol Head Neck Surg 1987;113:321–324.
24 Blake KD, Prasad C: CHARGE syndrome. Orphanet J Rare Dis 2006;1:34.
25 Zentner GE, Layman WS, Martin DM, Scacheri PC: Molecular and phenotypic aspects of CHD7 mutation in CHARGE syndrome. Am J Med Genet A 2010; 152A:674–686.
26 Lalani SR, Safiullah AM, Fernbach SD, et al: Spectrum of CHD7 mutations in 110 individuals with CHARGE syndrome and genotype-phenotype correlation. Am J Hum Genet 2006;78:303–314.
27 Powell CM, Michaelis RC: Townes-Brocks syndrome. J Med Genet 1999;36: 89–93.
28 O'Callaghan M, Young ID: The Townes-Brocks syndrome. J Med Genet 1990;27: 457–461.
29 Botzenhart EM, Green A, Ilyina H, et al: SALL1 mutation analysis in Townes-Brocks syndrome: twelve novel mutations and expansion of the phenotype. Hum Mutat 2005;26:282.
30 Smith RS, Zabaleta A, Kume T, Savinova OV, Kidson SH, Martin JE, Nishimura DY, Alward WL, Hogan BL, John SW: Haploinsufficiency of the transcription factors FOXC1 and FOXC2 results in aberrant ocular development. Hum Mol Genet 2000;9:1021–1032.
31 van der Burgt I: Noonan syndrome. Orphanet J Rare Dis 2007;2:4.
32 Schubbert S, Bollag G, Shannon K: Deregulated Ras signaling in developmental disorders: new tricks for an old dog. Curr Opin Genet Dev 2007;17: 15–22.
33 Cremers CW, van der Burgt CJ: Hearing loss in Noonan syndrome. Int J Pediatr Otorhinolaryngol 1992;23:81–84.
34 Sznajer Y, Keren B, Baumann C, Pereira S, Alberti C, Elion J, Cave H, Verloes A: The spectrum of cardiac anomalies in Noonan syndrome as a result of mutations in the PTPN11 gene. Pediatrics 2007;119:e1325–e1331.
35 Tidyman WE, Rauen KA: The RASopathies: developmental syndromes of Ras/MAPK pathway dysregulation. Curr Opin Genet Dev 2009;19:230–236.
36 Goldenberg I, Moss AJ, Zareba W, McNitt S, Robinson JL, Qi M, Towbin JA, Ackerman MJ, Murphy L: Clinical course and risk stratification of patients affected with the Jervell and Lange-Nielsen syndrome. J Cardiovasc Electrophysiol 2006;17:1161–1168.
37 Duggal P, Vesely MR, Wattanasirichaigoon D, Villafane J, Kaushik V, Beggs AH: Mutation of the gene for IsK associated with both Jervell and Lange-Nielsen and Romano-Ward forms of Long-QT syndrome. Circulation 1998;97:142–146.
38 Sarkozy A, Digilio MC, Dallapiccola B: Leopard syndrome. Orphanet J Rare Dis 2008;3:13.
39 Limongelli G, Pacileo G, Marino B, Digilio MC, Sarkozy A, Elliott P, Versacci P, Calabro P, De Zorzi A, Di Salvo G, Syrris P, Patton M, McKenna WJ, Dallapiccola B, Calabro R: Prevalence and clinical significance of cardiovascular abnormalities in patients with the LEOPARD syndrome. Am J Cardiol 2007;100:736–741.
40 Limongelli G, Sarkozy A, Pacileo G, Calabro P, Digilio MC, Maddaloni V, Gagliardi G, Di Salvo G, Iacomino M, Marino B, Dallapiccola B, Calabro R: Genotype-phenotype analysis and natural history of left ventricular hypertrophy in LEOPARD syndrome. Am J Med Genet A 2008;146A: 620–628.
41 Tartaglia M, Gelb BD: Noonan syndrome and related disorders: genetics and pathogenesis. Annu Rev Genomics Hum Genet 2005;6:45–68.
42 Digilio MC, Conti E, Sarkozy A, Mingarelli R, Dottorini T, Marino B, Pizzuti A, Dallapiccola B: Grouping of multiple-lentigines/LEOPARD and Noonan syndromes on the PTPN11 gene. Am J Hum Genet 2002;71:389–394.
43 Sarkozy A, Carta C, Moretti S, et al: Germline BRAF mutations in Noonan, LEOPARD, and cardiofaciocutaneous syndromes: molecular diversity and associated phenotypic spectrum. Hum Mutat 2009;30:695–702.
44 Pandit B, Sarkozy A, Pennacchio LA, et al: Gain-of-function RAF1 mutations cause Noonan and LEOPARD syndromes with hypertrophic cardiomyopathy. Nat Genet 2007;39:1007–1012.
45 Welsh LW: Alstrom syndrome: progressive deafness and blindness. Ann Otol Rhinol Laryngol 2007;116:281–285.
46 Marshall JD, Beck S, Maffei P, Naggert JK: Alstrom syndrome. Eur J Hum Genet 2007;15:1193–1202.
47 Weinstein R: Phytanic acid storage disease (Refsum's disease): clinical characteristics, pathophysiology and the role of therapeutic apheresis in its management. J Clin Apher 1999;14:181–184.
48 Kokotas H, Petersen MB, Willems PJ: Mitochondrial deafness. Clin Genet 2007;71:379–391.
49 Finsterer J: Genetic, pathogenetic, and phenotypic implications of the mitochondrial A3243G tRNALeu(UUR) mutation. Acta Neurol Scand 2007;116: 1–14.
50 Khanim F, Kirk J, Latif F, Barrett TG: WFS1/wolframin mutations, Wolfram syndrome, and associated diseases. Hum Mutat 2001;17:357–367.
51 Rigoli L, Lombardo F, Di Bella C: Wolfram syndrome and WFS1 gene. Clin Genet 2010 Aug 12 [Epub ahead of print].
52 Pijl S, Westerberg BD: Cochlear implantation results in patients with Kearns-Sayre syndrome. Ear Hear 2008;29:472–475.

53 Marin-Garcia J, Goldenthal MJ, Flores-Sarnat L, Sarnat HB: Severe mitochondrial cytopathy with complete A-V block, PEO, and mtDNA deletions. Pediatr Neurol 2002;27:213–216.

54 Gibson K, Halliday JL, Kirby DM, Yaplito-Lee J, Thorburn DR, Boneh A: Mitochondrial oxidative phosphorylation disorders presenting in neonates: clinical manifestations and enzymatic and molecular diagnoses. Pediatrics 2008;122:1003–1008.

55 Wold SM, Derkay CS, Darrow DH, Proud V: Role of the pediatric otolaryngologist in diagnosis and management of children with mucopolysaccharidoses. Int J Pediatr Otorhinolaryngol 2010;74:27–31.

56 Muenzer J, Wraith JE, Clarke LA: Mucopolysaccharidosis I: management and treatment guidelines. Pediatrics 2009;123:19–29.

57 Bonita RE, Cohen IS, Berko BA: Valvular heart disease in osteogenesis imperfecta: presentation of a case and review of the literature. Echocardiography 2010;27:69–73.

John W. Belmont, MD, PhD
Departments of Molecular and Human Genetics, and Pediatrics
Children's Nutrition Research Center
1100 Bates, Room 8070, Houston, TX 77030 (USA)
Tel. +1 713 798 4634, Fax +1 713 798 7187, E-Mail jbelmont@bcm.edu

Alford RL, Sutton VR (eds): Medical Genetics in the Clinical Practice of ORL.
Adv Otorhinolaryngol. Basel, Karger, 2011, vol 70, pp 75–83

Hearing Loss Disorders Associated with Renal Disease

William J. Kimberling[a,b] · Nicolo Borsa[d] · Richard J.H. Smith[c]

[a]Genetics Center, Boys Town National Research Hospital, Omaha, Nebr., Departments of [b]Ophthalmology and Visual Sciences, and [c]Otolaryngology Head and Neck Surgery, University of Iowa Carver School of Medicine, Iowa City, Iowa, USA; [d]Laboratory of Medical Genetics, Fondazione IRCCS Ca'Granda-Ospedale Maggiore Policlinico, Mangiagalli e Regina Elena, Milan, Italy

Abstract

There are several syndromes in which both hearing and renal function are impaired. The two best known are branchio-oto-renal (BOR) syndrome and Alport syndrome. These are reviewed along with several other rarer syndromes. BOR is especially important since it is likely to be first recognized by the otolaryngologist because of the hearing and branchial anomalies. It is important for the practicing otolaryngologist to recognize these disorders and to ensure that renal problems are being treated. In addition, the syndromes discussed here are all hereditary and referral to a clinical geneticist may be helpful to the individual and family.

There are developmental and physiological connections between the ear and the kidney as demonstrated by the fact that pathogenic mutations in several genes can deleteriously affect the function of both. The natures of these connections are not fully understood. Unlike the Usher syndromes (deaf-blindness), where it now appears that the nine Usher proteins form a single network called the interactome [1]. Genes involved in combined hearing and renal disorders appear to act in at least two unrelated ways. First, the kidney and ear share common transcription factors that contribute to the control of their development. Secondly, both the kidney and ear have highly developed and related strategies for the regulation of a normal ionic balance. While several hereditary hearing loss disorders are associated with renal problems, two appear frequently enough that the average otolaryngologist can expect to encounter affected patients. It is important therefore to recognize those hearing-impaired patients who may have significant renal disease. The various hearing loss disorders with accompanying renal problems discussed here are summarized in table 1.

Branchio-Oto-Renal Syndrome

Clinical Diagnosis

Branchio-oto-renal syndrome (BOR), a developmental disorder first described by Melnick et al. [2], has characteristic branchial, otologic and renal anomalies. The clinical diagnosis, based on criteria set by Chang et al. [3], requires the presence of three major or two major plus two minor findings, as shown in table 2. A single major anomaly is sufficient for the diagnosis if a first-degree relative is also affected.

Table 1. A listing of hearing-renal disorders for which the associated gene has been identified

Disease	OMIM	Gene	Genetics	Description
Branchio-oto-renal syndrome 1 (BOR1)	113650	*EYA1*	AD	hearing loss, preauricular pits, ear malformations, branchial anomalies, and renal anomalies
Branchio-oto-renal syndrome 2 (BOR2)	610896	*SIX5*	AD	
Branchio-otic syndrome 3 (BOS3)	601205	*SIX1*	AD	hearing loss, preauricular pits, ear malformations, branchial anomalies, and no renal anomalies
Townes-Brock syndrome	10748	*SALL1*	AD	Townes-Brocks syndrome (imperforate anus, triphalangial thumbs, and other anomalies of the hands and feet, and variable sensorineural hearing loss) plus occasionally preauricular pits, malformed ears, and hypoplastic kidneys
Alport syndrome		*COL4A5* *COL4A4* *COL4A3*	XL AR AR	nephritis and progressive hearing loss
Epstein syndrome	153650	*MYH9*	AD	macrothrombocytopenia, nephritis, and deafness
Muckle-Wells syndrome	191900	*NLRP3*	AD	uticaria, arthralgias, recurrent fever, late onset hearing loss, and renal amyloidosis
Renal tubular acidosis	267300	*ATP6B!*	AR	growth retardation, distal renal tubular acidosis, and hearing loss
Bartter syndrome IV	602522	*BSND*	AR	hypokalemic metabolic alkalosis and hearing loss
Papillorenal syndrome	120330	*PAX2*	AD	retinal and optic nerve coloboma; renal hypoplasia; vesicoureteral reflux; high frequency HL

OMIM stand for Online Mendelian Inheritance in Man that can provide a useful, up-to-date, understandable, and curated synopsis of all single genetic disorders in humans. It can be freely accessed at www.ncbi.nlm.nih.gov/omim/

There has been mild controversy over the inclusion of patients who have some but not all cardinal symptoms. Branchio-otic (BOS) and earpits-hearing-loss syndrome have been considered independent syndromes, however studies of the clinical variation in patients with *EYA1* pathogenic variants have documented a wide range of anomalies associated with variation within the *EYA1* gene on chromosome 8 [4]. Similarly, there are a number of genetic syndromes, such as CHARGE syndrome, where most individuals would meet the diagnostic

Table 2. Major and minor diagnostic criteria for branchio-oto-renal syndrome

Major criteria	Minor criteria
Second branchial arch anomalies	External auditory canal anomalies
Hearing loss	Middle ear anomalies
Preauricular pits	Inner ear anomalies
Auricular deformity	Preauricular tags
Renal anomalies	Facial asymmetry or palate anomalies

criteria for BOR but actually have a different syndrome.

About 75% of BOR patients have a hearing loss, though the extent and type of hearing loss varies considerably.

If hearing loss is present, severity may range from mild to profound in degree. Time of onset can be prelingual or late in onset, though usually before the end of the third decade [9]. While patients may not complain of vestibular symptoms, one study has shown that caloric responses are frequently reduced or abolished [5]. The cochlea may show a Mondini deformity and dysplasia of the horizontal semi-circular canal and an enlarged vestibular aqueduct can also be seen [10].

The external ears are often, but not invariably, abnormal: the abnormality can range from severe microtia to minor anomalies of the pinnae [6]. The middle ear also often presents with variable abnormality: the external canal may be atretic or stenotic and the ossicles may be malformed [2, 5, 6]. Cholesteatoma has been observed.

Branchial fistulae are present in about 60% of patients and usually appear as small openings anterior to the sternocleidomastoid muscle in the lower 1/3rd of the neck [9]. Fistulae occasionally track to the tonsillar fossae, and may drain and become infected; surgical excision is curative. Less frequently, a cyst may be palpable just deep to the sternocleidomastoid muscle at the level of the hyoid bone. Since both branchial clefts and fistulae are infrequently associated with other disorders, the presence of either should alert the clinician to the possibility of BOR. Minor anomalies associated with BOR in the facial area are aplastic or stenotic tear ducts [5, 11], palatal anomalies [6] and facial nerve paresis or paralysis [5, 9].

Renal anomalies have been reported to occur in about 80% of those carrying a EYA1 gene mutation [5, 9]. The kidneys may be normal, malpositioned, U-shaped, small or absent; duplication of the collecting systems has been reported [11, 12]. Agenesis of the kidneys occurs in about ~0.5% of all affected individuals and leads to Potter sequence and early infant death [13, 14]. Young parents at risk for transmitting BOR should be alerted to the possibility of having a newborn with lethal kidney problems. While the risk is small, the impact can be devastating. Renal agenesis can be diagnosed by fetal ultrasound.

Inheritance

BOR is inherited as an autosomal-dominant condition. There is no sex predilection in terms of frequency or severity. Given the extreme variability of the associated anomalies, it is important to consider the family history with regard to the diagnosis. For example, a family with a parent having malformed kidneys but no hearing loss or branchial anomaly whose child has malformed ears, hearing loss, and cervical cysts might well be considered to have BOR. This example underscores the fact that BOR is a 'family' disorder and diagnosis must take into account the phenotypes of the whole family and how they are transmitted. A mock BOR family is presented in pedigree form in figure 1 to illustrate this variability.

There are also a substantial number of patients with apparent BOR syndrome with no family history. These sporadic cases may be due to new mutations in *EYA1* and other BOR-associated genes, but may also represent a recessive form of the disorder or could be due to the extreme variable expressivity of BOR. The estimated prevalence of

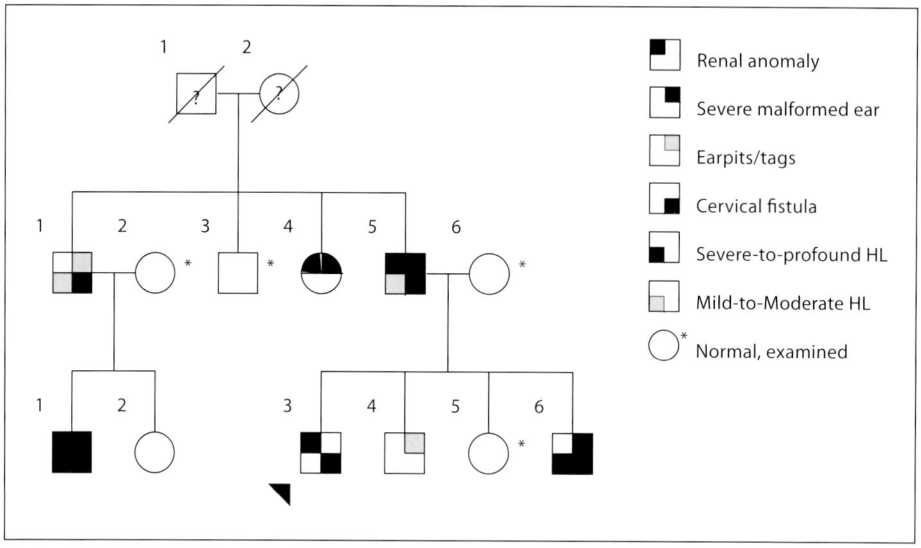

Fig. 1. Mock pedigree constructed from data in four different BOR families done to protect their privacy. The extreme variability is obvious and does typically occur even within families. Note that it is not known whether either of the grandparents in generation 1 is affected, a not uncommon observation due to expected unreliable information from older generations. Also, note individual 4 in generation three who only has ear pits. Ear pits are a minor anomaly and would be an insufficient finding upon which a clinical diagnosis could be made; DNA studies would be needed to be certain. Why there is such extreme variability is not yet well known. HL = Hearing loss.

BOR is 1/40,000 and occurs in about 2% of profoundly deaf children [13].

Genetic Causes

The first gene to be identified as causative for BOR was *EYA1* [15–17]. This gene was originally found in drosophila where mutations cause an eyeless phenotype. In humans, *EYA1* is the orthologue to the drosophila gene but it appears to have a greater role in branchial development and little, if any, role in the development of the eye.

In a recent study, 30–40% of the patients with a BOR phenotype were observed to have a pathogenic mutation in *EYA1* [4], but in patients who do not meet the BOR criteria, this figure falls to 20%. These mutations included both nonsense (large and small deletions, insertions, stops) and missense mutations. Approximately 2% of cases of BOR syndrome are due to mutations in *SIX1* and *SIX5* [18, 19].

DNA sequencing of *EYA1*, *SIX1* and *SIX5* provides a means of molecularly establishing a gene-specific BOR diagnosis. There are only a few laboratories that offer such testing as a clinical service. The reader is referred to GENETESTS at (http://www.ncbi.nlm.nih.gov/sites/GeneTests) to find a listing of which laboratories offer such testing.

The *EYA1*, *SIX1*, and *SIX5* proteins cooperate to activate the *SALL1* promoter [20]. Two families with mutations in *SALL1* have a BOR-like phenotype and lack some of the characteristics of Townes-Brocks syndrome that are more typical of mutations in this gene [21–23].

Since BOR syndrome is likely to come first to the attention of the otolaryngologist, we must be able to recognize the syndrome and make the appropriate referral to a nephrologist. Since BOR is inherited, a referral to a clinical geneticist or genetic counselor should be also be considered.

Treatment
Treatment consists of surgical excision of branchial anomalies. The hearing loss can be treated surgically or with hearing aids or cochlear implants, depending upon the type of malformation and the overall severity of the hearing loss. Renal symptoms may require treatment and on occasion, transplantation. The options for family planning for at risk parents are pre-implantation diagnosis and prenatal diagnosis.

Alport Syndrome

Clinical Diagnosis
Alport syndrome occurs with a frequency of 1/5,000 and is seen in about 1% of all children with childhood deafness [24]. It is a genetically heterogeneous disorder characterized by progressive nephritis that often leads to end-stage renal disease (ESRD). The hearing loss is progressive and sensorineural [25]. Three of the following criteria should be present to make a diagnosis of Alport syndrome: (1) positive family history of hematuria, chronic renal failure or both; (2) electron-microscopic evidence on renal biopsy; (3) characteristic ophthalmologic signs, i.e. anterior lenticonus and/or white macular flecks, and (4) high-frequency sensorineural hearing loss [26]. In addition, one should add the presence of a pathogenic mutation in one of the three genes associated with Alport syndrome.

X-linked Alport has a juvenile and an adult form distinguished by the severity of renal symptoms. The juvenile form, as expected from the name, has early-onset hematuria often presenting in infant boys as red diapers. The adult form is milder and reaches ESRD after 30 or more years [27, 28]. Nephrotic syndrome occurs in about half of cases [29], with hypertension beginning in the second decade. In males, the severity of symptoms may depend on the nature of the mutation [30], while in females the disease tends to be mild due to random X-chromosome inactivation which would predict expression of 50% normal protein. In the autosomal-recessive forms, both males and females progress to ESRD by about age 20; heterozygous carriers may exhibit mild renal symptoms [31].

The ophthalmologic findings characteristic of Alport syndrome include anterior lenticonus, macular flicks and peripheral coalescing flecks. Of these finding, lenticonus is considered by some investigators to be diagnostic of Alport syndrome [32].

Inheritance
For the practicing otolaryngologist who is suspicious of Alport syndrome, the family history can be a quick method of confirming, or at least heightening, one's suspicion. The most common mode of inheritance for both juvenile and adult Alport syndrome is X-linked. The presence of other affected males connected through the maternal line is consistent with this type of inheritance. For example, if a teenage male patient with a progressive sensorineural hearing loss has a maternal uncle who has had a renal transplant, Alport syndrome would be high on the differential diagnosis and referrals to nephrology and genetics are warranted.

Genetic Causes
Alport syndrome is a basement membrane disease involving type IV collagen. Collagen IV is a major component of all basement membranes and there are six genetically distinct collagen IV α chains, α1(IV)–α6(IV). The collagen α1(IV) and α2(IV) chains are the classical chains and are essentially ubiquitous in all basement membranes. Mutations in *COL4A1* and *COL4A2* have not been found and would likely cause embryonic

lethality. In contrast, the underlying genetic defect in Alport syndrome is mutation in one of three genes encoding type IV collagen chains 3, 4 and 5 [33]. These three chains have a restricted tissue distribution and are major components of the basement membranes of the glomerulus and cochlea [34, 35]. The more common X-linked Alport syndrome is caused by mutations in the collagen α5(IV) chain gene *COL4A5*; mutations in *COL4A3* and *COL4A4* are responsible for the autosomal forms of the disease [33, 36, 37].

Mutations affecting only one of the *COL4A3-COL4A5* genes result in the absence of all three gene products from the basement membrane since the α3–α5(IV) chains co-assemble in a manner that requires all three chains [38]. The non-mutated genes are translated normally, but the chains they encode are degraded once they fail to assemble due to the absence of a normal third chain.

COL4A5 is occasionally involved in a large deletion with adjacent genes. When the *COLA6* gene is included, Alport syndrome is associated with leiomyomatosis [39] and other anomalies [40].

Treatment
Current treatment of Alport syndrome must address the ESRD with dialysis or transplantation and the hearing loss with hearing aids or cochlear implantation. In the future, treatment may involve gene therapy [41, 42] although the development of antibodies against a new antigen in the kidney, as happens with kidney transplantation [43], may complicate this approach.

Miscellaneous Syndromes

Papillorenal Syndrome
Papillorenal syndrome shares some similarities to BOR syndrome. It presents with optic nerve anomalies, renal disease and hearing loss. The kidney disease can vary from lethal prenatal hypoplasia to asymptomatic proteinuria to normal renal development and function [44, 45]. The hearing loss usually involves the high frequencies but is not present in all patients [46, 47]. Optic disc coloboma is common and retinal and iris colobomas have been reported [48, 49]. It is caused by mutations in the *PAX2* transcription factor [47] and is inherited as an autosomal dominant with variable expression.

Epstein Syndrome
Epstein syndrome [50] is an autosomal-disorder due to pathogenic variation in the *MYH9* gene that encodes a nonmuscle myosin. It is an Alport-like disorder with megathrombocytopathy with or without nephritis and hearing loss, depending on the mutation location. Hematologic abnormalities are most frequently seen but mutation specifically in the myosin 9 motor domain results in an Alport-like phenotype [51, 52].

Muckle-Wells Syndrome
Muckle-Wells syndrome [53] is due to mutations in the *NLRP3* gene, which encodes a protein called cryopyrin. Cryopyrin belongs to the family of nucleotide-binding domain and leucine-rich repeat containing (NLR) proteins found in the cytoplasm of leukocytes and chondrocytes and is involved in inflammatory and immune responses [54, 55]. Mutations in *NLRP3* can cause familial cold autoinflammatory syndrome (uticaria, episodic fever, athropathy) with progressive sensorineural hearing loss and renal amyloidosis. The hearing loss starts in childhood progressing to severe to profound by the 4th decade of life.

Primary Renal Tubular Acidosis
Primary renal tubular acidosis [56] with hearing loss is an autosomal-recessive disorder due to mutations in the B1 subunit of H^+-ATPase, a proton pump protein present in the cochlea, endolymphatic sac and distal nephron [57]. The first presenting symptoms are failure to thrive, growth retardation and renal acidosis. Prognosis is good provided the disease is diagnosed and treated early. The hearing

loss is usually severe to profound and but has occasionally been reported to be progressive. It occurs in 87% of patients with pathogenic mutation in *ATP6B1* and does not respond to the alkali treatment used for the acidosis. Enlarged vestibular aqueducts have been observed [58–60].

Bartter Syndrome

Bartter Syndrome IV is an autosomal-recessive disorder due to mutations in the *BSND* gene that codes for barttin, an essential beta subunit for the CLC-Ka and CLC-Kb chloride channels [61, 62]. Furthermore, simultaneous mutations in both *CLCNKA* and *CLCNKB* genes are responsible for a *BSND*-like phenotype due to an apparent digenic effect [63]. Both the defects are associated with severe renal salt wasting, prelingual profound hearing loss and motor delay, the latter mainly occurs in patients with barttin defects. There is likely to be vestibular component to the motor delay since bartten is expressed in the crista ampullaris [61]. Good results are obtained with cochlear implants [64].

Conclusion

Progress in the last two decades has resulted in the identification of many genes associated with renal disease and hearing loss and it is expected that the number will increase. Not only do these discoveries yield insight into the common development and metabolic connections between the ear and the kidney, they also improve the diagnosis, and thus the management, of these conditions. A correct molecular diagnosis combined with thorough clinical evaluation will help with treatment, prognosis and genetic counseling. Otolaryngologists should be familiar with BOR syndrome and Alport syndrome. In addition to these two common syndromes and the rarer syndromes discussed in this chapter, there are numerous disorders in which renal disease is associated with hearing loss but where the causative gene is unknown [65]. For all of these syndromes, the otolaryngologist in encouraged to seek the help of clinical geneticists and nephrologists to optimize patient care.

References

1 Reiners J, Nagel-Wolfrum K, Jurgens K, Marker T, Wolfrum U: Molecular basis of human Usher syndrome: deciphering the meshes of the Usher protein network provides insights into the pathomechanisms of the Usher disease. Exp Eye Res 2006;83:97–119.

2 Melnick M, Bixler D, Nance WE, Silk K, Yune H: Familial branchio-oto-renal dysplasia: a new addition to the branchial arch syndromes. Clin Genet 1976;9:25–34.

3 Chang EH, Menezes M, Meyer NC, et al: Branchio-oto-renal syndrome: the mutation spectrum in EYA1 and its phenotypic consequences. Hum Mutat 2004;23:582–589.

4 Orten DJ, Fischer SM, Sorensen JL, et al: Branchio-oto-renal syndrome (BOR): novel mutations in the EYA1 gene, and a review of the mutational genetics of BOR. Hum Mutat 2008;29:537–544.

5 Cremers CWRJ, Fikkers-Van Noord M: The earpits-deafness syndrome: clinical and genetic aspects. Int J Pediatr Otorhinolaryngol 1980;2:309–322.

6 Fraser FC, Ling D, Clogg D, Nogrady B: Genetic aspects of the BOR syndrome – branchial fistulas, ear pits, hearing loss, and renal anomalies. Am J Med Genet 1978;2:241–252.

7 Cremers CWRJ, Thijssen HOM, Fischer AJEM, Marres EHMA: Otological aspects of the earpit-deafness syndrome. ORL 1981;43:223–239.

8 Fitch N, Lindsay JR, Srolovitz H: The temporal bone in the preauricular pit, cervical fistula, hearing loss syndrome. Ann Otol 1976;85:268–275.

9 Chen A, Francis M, Ni L, et al: Phenotypic manifestations of branchio-oto-renal syndrome. Am J Med Genet 1995;58:365–370.

10 Ceruti S, Stinckens C, Cremers CW, Casselman JW: Temporal bone anomalies in the branchio-oto-renal syndrome: detailed computed tomographic and magnetic resonance imaging findings. Otol Neurotol 2002;23:200–207.

11 Heimler A, Lieber E: BOR syndrome: reduced penetrance and variable expressivity in 4 generations of a large kindred. Am J Med Genet 1986;25:15–27.

12 Fraser FC, Ayme S, Halal F, Sproule JR: Autosomal dominant duplication of the renal collecting system, hearing loss, and external ear anomalies: a new syndrome? Am J Med Gen 1983;14:473–478.

13 Fraser FC, Sproule JR, Halal F: Frequency of the branchio-oto-renal (BOR) syndrome in children with profound hearing loss. Am J Med Genet 1980;7:341–349.

14 Raspino M, Tarantino V, Moni L, Verrina E, Ciardi MR, Gusmano R: The branchio-oto-renal syndrome: report of 2 family groups. J Laryngol Otol 1988; 102:138–141.
15 Abdelhak S, Kalatzis V, Heilig R, et al: Clustering of mutations responsible for branchio-oto-renal (BOR) syndrome in the eyes absent homologous region (eyaHR) of EYA1. Hum Mol Genet 1997; 6:2247–2255.
16 Abdelhak S, Kalatzis V, Heilig R, et al: A human homologue of the Drosophila eyes absent gene underlies branchio-oto-renal (BOR) syndrome and identifies a novel gene family. Nat Genet 1997;15: 157–164.
17 Smith RJ, Coppage KB, Ankerstjerne JK, et al: Localization of the gene for branchiootorenal syndrome to chromosome 8q. Genomics 1992;14:841–844.
18 Hoskins BE, Cramer CH, Silvius D, et al: Transcription factor SIX5 is mutated in patients with branchio-oto-renal syndrome. Am J Hum Genet 2007;80:800–804.
19 Ruf RG, Xu PX, Silvius D, et al: SIX1 mutations cause branchio-oto-renal syndrome by disruption of EYA1-SIX1-DNA complexes. Proc Natl Acad Sci USA 2004;101:8090–8095.
20 Chai L, Yang J, Di C, et al: Transcriptional activation of the SALL1 by the human SIX1 homeodomain during kidney development. J Biol Chem 2006;281:18918–18926.
21 Albrecht B, Liebers M, Kohlhase J: Atypical phenotype and intrafamilial variability associated with a novel SALL1 mutation. Am J Med Gen 2004;125A: 102–104.
22 Engels S, Kohlhase J, McGaughran J: A SALL1 mutation causes a branchio-oto-renal syndrome-like phenotype. J Med Genet 2000;37:458–460.
23 Botzenhart EM, Bartalini G, Blair E, et al: Townes-Brocks syndrome: twenty novel SALL1 mutations in sporadic and familial cases and refinement of the SALL1 hot spot region. Hum Mutat 2007;28:204–205.
24 Flinter F: Alport's syndrome: a clinical and genetic study. Contrib Nephrol. Basel, Karger, 1990, vol 80, pp 9–16.
25 Gleeson MJ: Alport's syndrome: audiological manifestations and implications. J Laryngol Otol 1984;98:449–465.
26 Flinter FA, Cameron JS, Chantler C, Houston I, Bobrow M: Genetics of classic Alport's syndrome. Lancet 1988;ii: 1005–1007.
27 Gubler MC, Antignac C, Deschenes G, et al: Genetic, clinical, and morphologic heterogeneity in Alport's syndrome. Adv Nephrol Necker Hosp 1993;22:15–35.
28 Gubler MC: Inherited diseases of the glomerular basement membrane. Nat Clin Pract Nephrol 2008;4:24–37.
29 Grunfeld JP, Charbonneau R, Grateau G, Noel LH: Alport's syndrome and related hereditary nephropathies. Contrib Nephrol. Basel, Karger, 1988, vol 61, pp 82–90.
30 Jais JP, Knebelmann B, Giatras I, et al: X-linked Alport syndrome: natural history and genotype-phenotype correlations in girls and women belonging to 195 families: a 'European Community Alport Syndrome Concerted Action' study. J Am Soc Nephrol 2003;14:2603–2610.
31 Thorner PS: Alport syndrome and thin basement membrane nephropathy. Nephron Clin Pract 2007;106:c82–c88.
32 Fawzi AA, Lee NG, Eliott D, Song J, Stewart JM: Retinal findings in patients with Alport syndrome: expanding the clinical spectrum. Br J Ophthalmol 2009; 93:1606–1611.
33 Barker DF, Hostikka SL, Zhou J, et al: Identification of mutations in the COL4A5 collagen gene in Alport syndrome. Science 1990;248:1224–1227.
34 Kleppel MM, Kashtan C, Santi PA, Wieslander J, Michael AF: Distribution of familial nephritis antigen in normal tissue and renal basement membranes of patients with homozygous and heterozygous Alport familial nephritis: relationship of familial nephritis and Goodpasture antigens to novel collagen chains and type IV collagen. Lab Invest 1989;61:278–289.
35 Kleppel MM, Fan WW, Cheong HI, Kashtan CE, Michael AF: Immunochemical studies of the Alport antigen. Kidney Int 1992;41:1629–1637.
36 Lemmink HH, Mochizuki T, van den Heuvel LP, et al: Mutations in the type IV collagen alpha 3 (COL4A3) gene in autosomal recessive Alport syndrome. Hum Mol Genet 1994;3:1269–1273.
37 Mochizuki T, Lemmink HH, Mariyama M, et al: Identification of mutations in the alpha 3(IV) and alpha 4(IV) collagen genes in autosomal recessive Alport syndrome. Nat Genet 1994;8:77–81.
38 Hudson BG, Reeders ST, Tryggvason K: Type IV collagen: structure, gene organization, and role in human diseases: molecular basis of Goodpasture and Alport syndromes and diffuse leiomyomatosis. J Biol Chem 1993;268:26033–26036.
39 Garcia-Torres R, Cruz D, Orozco L, Heidet L, Gubler MC: Alport syndrome and diffuse leiomyomatosis: clinical aspects, pathology, molecular biology and extracellular matrix studies. A synthesis. Nephrologie 2000;21:9–12.
40 Piccini M, Vitelli F, Bruttini M, et al: FACL4, a new gene encoding long-chain acyl-CoA synthetase 4, is deleted in a family with Alport syndrome, elliptocytosis, and mental retardation. Genomics 1998;47:350–358.
41 Gross O, Kashtan CE: Treatment of Alport syndrome: beyond animal models. Kidney Int 2009;76:599–603.
42 Imai E, Isaka Y: Perspectives for gene therapy in renal diseases. Intern Med 2004;43:85–96.
43 Kashtan CE: Renal transplantation in patients with Alport syndrome. Pediatr Transplant 2006;10:651–657.
44 Eccles MR, Schimmenti LA: Renal-coloboma syndrome: a multi-system developmental disorder caused by PAX2 mutations. Clin Genet 1999;56:1–9.
45 Ford B, Rupps R, Lirenman D, et al: Renal-coloboma syndrome: prenatal detection and clinical spectrum in a large family. Am J Med Genet 2001;99: 137–141.
46 Schimmenti LA, Cunliffe HE, McNoe LA, et al: Further delineation of renal-coloboma syndrome in patients with extreme variability of phenotype and identical *PAX2* mutations. Am J Hum Genet 1997;60:869–878.
47 Sanyanusin P, Schimmenti LA, McNoe LA, et al: Mutation of the PAX2 gene in a family with optic nerve colobomas, renal anomalies and vesicoureteral reflux. Nat Genet 1995;9:358–364.
48 Amiel J, Audollent S, Joly D, et al: PAX2 mutations in renal-coloboma syndrome: mutational hotspot and germline mosaicism. Eur J Hum Genet 2000;8:820–826.
49 Dureau P, Attie-Bitach T, Salomon R, et al: Renal coloboma syndrome. Ophthalmology 2001;108:1912–1916.
50 Epstein CJ, Sahud MA, Piel CF, et al: Hereditary macrothrombocytopathia, nephritis and deafness. Am J Med 1972; 52:299–310.

51 Pecci A, Canobbio I, Balduini A, et al: Pathogenetic mechanisms of hematological abnormalities of patients with MYH9 mutations. Hum Mol Genet 2005;14:3169–3178.
52 Pecci A, Panza E, Pujol-Moix N, et al: Position of nonmuscle myosin heavy chain IIA (NMMHC-IIA) mutations predicts the natural history of MYH9-related disease. Hum Mutat 2008;29:409–417.
53 Muckle TJ, Wells SM: Urticaria, deafness, and amyloidosis: a new heredofamilial syndrome. Q J Med 1962;31:235–248.
54 Aganna E, Martinon F, Hawkins PN, et al: Association of mutations in the NALP3/CIAS1/PYPAF1 gene with a broad phenotype including recurrent fever, cold sensitivity, sensorineural deafness, and AA amyloidosis. Arthritis Rheum 2002;46:2445–2452.
55 Aganna E, Hawkins PN, Ozen S, et al: Allelic variants in genes associated with hereditary periodic fever syndromes as susceptibility factors for reactive systemic AA amyloidosis. Genes Immun 2004;5:289–293.
56 Cohen T, Brand-Auraban A, Karshai C, et al: Familial infantile renal tubular acidosis and congenital nerve deafness: an autosomal recessive syndrome. Clin Genet 1973;4:275–278.
57 Karet FE, Finberg KE, Nelson RD, et al: Mutations in the gene encoding B1 subunit of H^+-ATPase cause renal tubular acidosis with sensorineural deafness. Nat Genet 1999;21:84–90.
58 Berrettini S, Forli F, Bogazzi F, et al: Large vestibular aqueduct syndrome: audiological, radiological, clinical, and genetic features. Am J Otolaryngol 2005;26:363–371.
59 Berrettini S, Neri E, Forli F, et al: Large vestibular aqueduct in distal renal tubular acidosis: high-resolution MR in three cases. Acta Radiol 2001;42:320–322.
60 Andreucci E, Bianchi B, Carboni I, et al: Inner ear abnormalities in four patients with dRTA and SNHL: clinical and genetic heterogeneity. Pediatr Nephrol 2009;24:2147–2153.
61 Birkenhager R, Otto E, Schurmann MJ, et al: Mutation of BSND causes Bartter syndrome with sensorineural deafness and kidney failure. Nat Genet 2001;29:310–314.
62 Landau D, Shalev H, Ohaly M, Carmi R: Infantile variant of Bartter syndrome and sensorineural deafness: a new autosomal recessive disorder. Am J Med Genet 1995;59:454–459.
63 Schlingmann KP, Konrad M, Jeck N, et al: Salt wasting and deafness resulting from mutations in two chloride channels. N Engl J Med 2004;350:1314–1319.
64 Jeck N, Reinalter SC, Henne T, et al: Hypokalemic salt-losing tubulopathy with chronic renal failure and sensorineural deafness. Pediatrics 2001;108:E5.
65 Bitner-Glindzicz M, Heath KE, Campos-Barros A: Genetic hearing loss associated with renal disorders; in Toriello HV, Reardon W, Gorlin RJ (eds): Hereditary Hearing Loss and its Syndromes, ed 2. New York, Oxford University Press, 2004, pp 267–289.

William J. Kimberling
Boys Town Research Hospital
555 North 30th Street
Omaha, NE 68131 (USA)
E-Mail William.Kimberling@boystown.org

Alford RL, Sutton VR (eds): Medical Genetics in the Clinical Practice of ORL.
Adv Otorhinolaryngol. Basel, Karger, 2011, vol 70, pp 84–90

Multiple Endocrine Neoplasia: Types 1 and 2

Deborah J. Marsh[a] · Oliver Gimm[b,c]

[a]Hormones and Cancer Group, Kolling Institute of Medical Research, Royal North Shore Hospital, University of Sydney E25, St. Leonards, N.S.W., Australia; [b]Department of Surgery and [c]Institute for Clinical and Experimental Medicine (IKE), University Hospital, Linköping, Sweden

Abstract

Multiple endocrine neoplasia type 1 (MEN 1) and type 2 (MEN 2) are autosomal-dominantly inherited syndromes where highly penetrant germline mutations predispose patients to the development of tumours in hormone-secreting cells. In the case of MEN 1, loss-of-function germline mutations in the tumour suppressor gene *MEN1* increase the risk of developing pituitary, parathyroid and pancreatic islet tumours, and less commonly thymic carcinoids, lipomas and benign adrenocortical tumours. In the case of MEN 2, gain-of-function germline mutations clustered in specific codons of the *RET* proto-oncogene increase the risk of developing medullary thyroid carcinoma (MTC), phaeochromocytoma and parathyroid tumours. Offering *RET* testing is best practice for the clinical management of patients at-risk of MEN 2, and MEN 2 has become a classic model for the integration of molecular medicine into patient care. Prophylactic thyroidectomy in an asymptomatic *RET* mutation carrier to address the risk of developing MTC can prevent or cure this malignancy. No similar preventative strategies can be employed to prevent or cure MEN 1-associated tumours. Genetic testing for MEN 1 is therefore both more complex due to a general lack of mutational hotspots, and the benefit to patients is less straight forward. While a number of genotype-phenotype correlations exist in MEN 2, providing further rationale for performing genetic testing in this condition, these correlations are absent in MEN 1. This review summarises our current knowledge of these two syndromes with emphasis on those aspects with specific relevance to the otorhinolaryngologist.

Multiple endocrine neoplasia (MEN) types 1 and 2 are part of a group of rare familial endocrine neoplasia disorders characterised by the presence of tumours in hormone secreting cells along with other disorders including von Hippel-Lindau disease, familial paraganglioma and phaeochromocytoma, Cowden syndrome, hyperparathyroidism jaw-tumour syndrome and Carney complex (reviewed in Marsh and Zori [1]). MEN 1 and MEN 2 fall at either end of the spectrum when considering both the ease of conducting genetic testing, and the ability to act on genetic information to prevent or cure a tumour.

Multiple Endocrine Neoplasia Type 1

Clinical Presentation/Phenotype

MEN 1 has been estimated to occur in between 1 in 10,000 to 1 in 100,000 people [2] and is characterised by neuroendocrine tumours of the gastro-enteric-pancreatic tract. These lesions include parathyroid tumours causing primary hyperparathyroidism (pHPT), pancreatic islet cell tumours, anterior pituitary tumours, and less commonly thymic carcinoids, lipomas, thyroid tumours, benign tumours of the adrenal cortex, and atypically generally benign tumours of the

Table 1. Clinical presentations of patients with MEN 1 and MEN 2

Organ	Type of tumour/disease	Biochemical investigation	Suggested age to commence screening, years
MEN 1			
Parathyroid	primary hyperparathyroidism	(ionised) calcium, (intact) parathormone	10
Pancreas	insulinoma	insulin, fasting glucose	5
	gastrinoma	(stimulated) gastrin	20
	other tumours	chromogranin A, pancreatic polypeptide, proinsulin, glucagon	20
Pituitary	prolactinoma	prolactin	?
Foregut	carcinoids	serotonin, 5-hydroxyindoleacetic acid (5-HIAA)	20
	thymic carcinoids	serotonin	20–25
MEN 2			
Thyroid	medullary thyroid carcinoma	calcitonin	MEN 2A: 5–10 MEN 2B: birth
Parathyroid	primary hyperparathyroidism	(ionised) calcium, (intact) parathormone	MEN 2A: 20–35 MEN 2B: never
Adrenal	phaeochromocytoma	catecholamines, metanephrines, vanillylmandelic acid (VMA), chromogranin A	30–40

adrenal medulla (phaeochromocytoma); however, presentation can vary markedly between two individuals (table 1).

Diagnostic criteria for MEN 1 specifies that an individual must have abnormalities in at least two of the more commonly affected endocrine glands, as well as a first-degree relative with at least one MEN 1-related lesion or a known *MEN1* mutation [3]. Almost 50% of MEN 1 patients will succumb to MEN 1-related disease, most frequently associated with pancreatic islet cell tumours [4]. Almost all patients with MEN 1 develop pHPT that can lead to hypercalcemia throughout their lifetime, and although this is almost always benign, its recurring nature can make surgical management difficult. In comparison to sporadic pHPT, these patients typically present between 20 and 25 years of age, approximately 30 years earlier than their sporadic counterparts [5]. Biochemical screening is recommended from the age of 10 years. The underlying genetic cause implies that all parathyroid glands can be affected. In fact, by the time of diagnosis, most patients already present with multiple parathyroid gland enlargement classified as either parathyroid hyperplasia or multiple adenomas. In MEN 1 patients, the diagnosis of pHPT is made if both parathyroid hormone (PTH) and ionised calcium levels are elevated [6].

Genetic Background/Genotype

Germline mutations in the tumour suppressor gene *MEN1* were first identified in 1997 in patients with MEN 1 [7, 8]. *MEN1* mutations are also found rarely in the related condition Familial Isolated Hyperparathyroidism (FIH). *MEN1* consists of 10 exons, where exon 1 is not translated. It encodes the 610 amino acid (67 kDa) ubiquitously expressed and predominantly nuclear protein menin that has roles in the regulation of transcription, controlling genome stability, the regulation of cell division and cell cycle control. Up to 90% of MEN 1 patients will have a *MEN1* mutation, with approximately 10% of these mutations appearing to be de novo, i.e. identified in patients with apparently sporadic parathyroid adenomas [9].

Mutations are predicted to be loss of function and include small (and less frequently large) deletions, small insertions, insertion-deletions, as well as nonsense and missense point mutations and splicing mutations, with the majority predicted to prematurely truncate menin [10, 11]. There are over 570 mutation entries for *MEN1* in The Human Genome Mutation Database, Cardiff, UK (http://www.hgmd.cf.ac.uk/ac/index.php), and well over 1,000 mutations reported in total [11], with mutations covering the entirety of the gene. There is some indication of potential mutational hot-spots at codons 83–84, 516 and 210–211 accounting for approximately 12% of all mutations [11]; however, in general, lack of frequent mutational clusters complicates genetic screening for this disorder. Of note, in MEN 1 patients without *MEN1* mutation, germline mutations in one of the cyclin-dependent kinase inhibitor genes have been reported; however, these would appear to be rare [12].

Genotype-Phenotype Correlations

No appreciable genotype-phenotype correlations have been identified in MEN 1 [11, 13, 14].

Genetic Screening

Knowledge of a patient's *MEN1* mutation carrier status is useful for clinical management strategies and life-planning decisions, but cannot avoid or cure the malignancies associated with this condition [3]. This is largely because there are no options for prophylactic surgery for MEN 1 patients, who are generally not treated until their condition first manifests. Biochemical screening to search for early disease in asymptomatic mutation carriers is recommended. If a member of a family tests negative for a *MEN1* mutation that is present in affected family members, this removes them from the lifelong burden of biochemical and radiological screening for associated tumours. Guidelines have been published outlining recommended diagnostic tests and therapy for *MEN1* mutation carriers [5, 10].

Surgery and Experimental Therapies

The indication to operate is given in any MEN 1 patient with the diagnosis of pHPT. Prior to primary surgery, sophisticated imaging techniques are generally not recommended since their sensitivity is low in MEN 1-associated pHPT [15]. Due to the fact that MEN 1-associated pHPT is a multiglandular disease, an attempt must be made to identify all parathyroid glands intraoperatively. This implies routine removal of the thyrothymic ligament where parathyroid glands can be found in up to 20% of patients. Once all parathyroid glands are localised, the smallest gland should be identified. A remnant about half the size of a normal gland should either be left in situ (referred to as subtotal parathyroidectomy) or be autotransplanted (referred to as total parathyroidectomy and autotransplantation). The other parathyroid glands shall be removed completely. As recurrence of the preserved tissue is common, if subtotal parathyroidectomy is performed the remnant should be marked with a non-absorbable suture or clip in order to facilitate reoperation [15].

Calcimimetics, calcium-sensing receptor agonists, show promise for the treatment of sporadic pHPT and may have a role in treating elevated PTH in the context of MEN 1 [5, 16, 17]. Depot long-acting octreotide has also been used to treat MEN 1-associated pHPT [18]. Multicentre, randomised clinical trials still need to be conducted in order to assess the efficacy of these experimental therapies.

Multiple Endocrine Neoplasia Type 2

Clinical Presentation/Phenotype

MEN 2 is believed to occur in 1 in 200,000 live births [19]. The clinical presentation of MEN 2 may vary significantly between two individuals and includes pHPT, medullary thyroid carcinoma (MTC; a malignant tumour of parafollicular thyroid C cells that secrete calcitonin) and phaeochromocytoma (phaeo; tumour of the adrenal medulla) (table 1). If two or more of these tumours are present in 1 patient or in a close relative, a diagnosis of MEN 2 should be considered. Around two thirds of people harbouring a *RET* mutation will develop one or more of these tumours by 70 years of age [20].

Clinically and genetically, two major types can be distinguished, namely MEN 2A and MEN 2B. In contrast to MEN 2A, patients with MEN 2B present with a Marfanoid habitus, mucosal neuromas (which often cause the lips to appear large and patulous) and ganglioneuromatosis of the gastrointestinal tract that are clues for this clinical diagnosis. A third form that is also part of the clinical and genetic MEN 2 spectrum is familial medullary thyroid carcinoma (FMTC) where MTC is the only phenotype, and often displays a later age of onset [5].

From the otorhinolaryngological point of view, MTC and pHPT are the two MEN 2-associated diseases that may need surgical treatment. Approximately 25% of all MTCs occur as part of MEN 2, with patients presenting at a younger age compared to their sporadic counterparts, particularly when identified as part of a family screening program. If not identified during family screening procedures, patients usually present with either a thyroid tumour and/or cervical lymph node metastases.

MEN 2-associated pHPT is seen in up to 30% of patients with MEN 2A, and may include hyperplasia or adenoma. pHPT is not reported in MEN 2B patients. Patients with MEN 2A-associated pHPT in general present with a very mild form of pHPT that is often asymptomatic. Severe manifestations are occasionally reported and, as is the case for MEN 1, MEN 2-associated parathyroid carcinoma is exceedingly rare. While the underlying genetic cause implies that all parathyroid glands may be affected in MEN 2, often only one gland is enlarged. Both Hirschsprung disease, a lack of enteric ganglia in the hindgut, and the skin disorder cutaneous lichen amyloidosis have been reported in MEN 2A/FMTC families [5].

Genetic Background/Genotype

Gain-of-function mutations in the proto-oncogene *RET* were first identified in the germline of patients with MEN 2A in 1993, making MEN 2 the first inherited endocrine neoplasia to be clarified at the molecular level [21]. Identification of *RET* mutations associated with MEN 2B and FMTC followed shortly thereafter (reviewed in Marsh et al. [22]). In the spectrum of familial cancer syndromes, activating mutations in a proto-oncogene are rare, with the vast majority of inherited cancer syndromes being caused by loss of function of a tumour-suppressor gene such as is seen in MEN 1 (reviewed in Marsh and Zori [1]). The RET gene codes for a transmembrane receptor tyrosine kinase with roles in proliferation, migration and differentiation of neural crest-derived tissue.

Although *RET* has 21 coding exons, MEN 2-associated germline mutations are essentially confined to 7 of these exons (exons 8, 10, 11, 13, 14, 15 and 16) and are almost exclusively missense mutations. Activating germline mutations in cysteines in *RET* exon 10 codons 609, 611, 618 or 620, and exon 11 codons 630 or 634 would appear to account for over 95% of MEN 2A families. Mutations are also found less frequently in non-cysteine residues, 768, 790, 791, 804 and 891, and predominantly in families with FMTC. Specific *RET* mutations account for MEN 2B; most commonly M918T in exon 16, and less frequently A883F in exon 15 (reviewed in Marsh et al. [22]). More than 50% of these MEN 2B mutations appear to be de novo.

Genotype-Phenotype Correlations

Genotype-phenotype correlations have been identified in MEN 2 by international multi-centre studies considering the family as a unit. These studies have indicated that the presence of a codon 634 mutation confers a higher risk of pHPT and phaeo [23, 24]. Specifically, presence of the C634R mutation has been reported to confer an even greater risk of pHPT than other mutations in the same codon [23], although this has not been shown for all studies. Furthermore, the C634R mutation has been reported to be associated with a higher incidence of metastases at diagnosis, while mutations at codon 634 have been associated with cutaneous lichen amyloidosis (reviewed in Wiesner and Snow-Bailey [25]). Families in which MEN 2A or FMTC co-segregate with Hirschsprung's disease tend to have germline *RET* mutations in codons 618 and 620 (reviewed in Eng [19]). Despite all of these correlations, it is important to observe that individuals within a single family who carry the same *RET* mutation can still display a highly variable phenotype.

Genetic Screening

Screening for *RET* mutations in patients either with MEN 2 or who are at-risk of developing this disease is recommended and suggested to be superior to the biochemical screening method for this disease that relies on the measurement of elevated calcitonin levels to detect the presence of MTC. As MTC can occur in very young children, it is suggested that *RET* testing should be performed at or before 5 years of age in at-risk children [5]. Given the clustering of mutations in certain codons, the development of screening programs that might involve methods such as direct sequencing, denaturing high-performance liquid chromatography, high resolution melt analysis, etc., is relatively straight forward. The benefits of genetic screening for MEN 2 are clear, in that prophylactic thyroidectomy can be performed in children with the ability to prevent or cure MTC. Knowledge of the exact *RET* mutation will give clues as to the likely aggressiveness of disease as indicated above, and can influence the age at which surgery is performed and perhaps even the extent of surgery.

Guidelines suggest that given the link between pHPT and codon 634 mutations, patients who harbour these mutations, and especially those with a C634R mutation, should be screened annually for pHPT by serum calcium and PTH testing [5].

Surgery and Experimental Therapies

In contrast to the sporadic form, MEN 2-associated MTC is a multifocal disease and thyroid tissue left in situ is prone to develop MTC. Thus, total thyroidectomy should be performed and thyroid hormone replacement therapy instigated. Due to the high prevalence of often small lymph node metastases (LNM), a central cervical lymph node dissection should be included in index patients, i.e. patients with clinically overt MTC, even if no LNM are found pre- or intraoperatively. In patients identified through *RET* mutation analysis, no central lymph node dissection is necessary if the calcitonin level is normal [26]. The onset of MTC in patients with MEN 2B is much earlier as compared to MEN 2A (table 1) and patients should be treated as soon as the diagnosis is made.

MEN 2A-associated pHPT is rarely evident before the patient undergoes surgery for MTC where the opportunity exists to assess all parathyroid glands for enlargement. Prior to surgery sophisticated imaging techniques for pHPT are generally not recommended. Despite the fact that MEN 2A-associated pHPT has an underlying genetic cause, multiglandular disease is rarely seen. Still, an attempt should be made to identify all parathyroid glands intraoperatively. Once all parathyroid glands are localised, only glands that are enlarged need be removed [6]. Routine autotransplantation of parathyroid tissue is not necessary. However, a normal parathyroid gland identified during surgery for MTC that appears to have compromised vascularity (darkening of its surface) should be autotransplanted and marked as described for MEN 1.

Molecular target drugs that inhibit tyrosine kinase activity and angiogenesis are being investigated as therapies for MEN 2, predominantly as a treatment for advanced or metastatic MTC. One such drug, vandetanib (ZD6474) that is an inhibitor of RET and epidermal growth factor receptor (also a tyrosine kinase) activity, as well as vascular endothelial growth factor receptor shows promise [27]. As we enter the era of personalised medicine based on the presence of specific mutations and other molecular events in patients, it is expected that additional options will arise for the treatment of MTC, pHPT and other manifestations of MEN 2.

Conclusions

In summary, genetic testing is recommended for at-risk individuals in both MEN 1 and MEN 2 families; however, the ability to surgically prevent or cure an inherited malignancy based on this molecular knowledge is currently only possible in MEN 2. Clinical cancer geneticists and genetic counsellors should be part of a multidisciplinary team in addition to endocrinologists, endocrine surgeons, and where relevant, endocrine paediatricians managing MEN patients and their families. As new molecular target drugs are discovered, knowledge of a patient's mutation status, and likely the precise mutation, will become increasingly more important. The call for patients to participate in multicentre, randomised clinical trials to assess the efficacy of these experimental therapies will likely increase in coming years. For further reading, recent reviews and reports are recommended that cover in more detail a number of topics raised in this chapter [10, 19, 22, 25].

Acknowledgements

D.J.M. is a Cancer Institute NSW Fellow (Australia).

References

1 Marsh D, Zori R: Genetic insights into familial cancers – update and recent discoveries. Cancer Lett 2002;181:125–164.
2 Kopp P: A long-sought needle in the haystack: the multiple endocrine neoplasia type 1 gene. Eur J Endocrinol 1997; 137:222–223.
3 Schussheim DH, Skarulis MC, Agarwal SK, Simonds WF, Burns AL, Spiegel AM, et al: Multiple endocrine neoplasia type 1: new clinical and basic findings. Trends Endocrinol Metab 2001;12: 173–178.
4 Doherty GM, Olson JA, Frisella MM, Lairmore TC, Wells SA Jr, Norton JA: Lethality of multiple endocrine neoplasia type I. World J Surg 1998;22:581–586;discussion 6–7.
5 Brandi ML, Gagel RF, Angeli A, et al: Guidelines for diagnosis and therapy of MEN type 1 and type 2. J Clin Endocrinol Metab 2001;86:5658–5671.
6 Sierra M, Gibelin H, Kraimps JL: Multiple endocrine neoplasia type 1; in Clark O, Duh Q-Y, Kebebew E (eds): Textbook of Endocrine Surgery. Philadelphia, Elsevier Saunders, 2005, pp 489–492.
7 Chandrasekharappa SC, Guru SC, Manickam P, et al: Positional cloning of the gene for multiple endocrine neoplasia-type 1. Science 1997;276: 404–407.
8 Lemmens I, Van de Ven WJ, Kas K, Zhang CX, Giraud S, Wautot V, et al: Identification of the multiple endocrine neoplasia type 1 (MEN1) gene: the European Consortium on MEN1. Hum Mol Genet 1997;6:1177–1183.
9 Chandrasekharappa SC, Teh BT: Functional studies of the MEN1 gene. J Intern Med 2003;253:606–615.
10 Falchetti A, Marini F, Brandi ML: Multiple endocrine neoplasia type 1. Gene Reviews. Seattle, University of Washington, 2010, pp 1–37.
11 Lemos MC, Thakker RV: Multiple endocrine neoplasia type 1 (MEN1): analysis of 1336 mutations reported in the first decade following identification of the gene. Hum Mutat 2008;29:22–32.

12 Agarwal SK, Mateo CM, Marx SJ: Rare germline mutations in cyclin-dependent kinase inhibitor genes in multiple endocrine neoplasia type 1 and related states. J Clin Endocrinol Metab 2009;94:1826–1834.
13 Giraud S, Zhang CX, Serova-Sinilnikova O, et al: Germ-line mutation analysis in patients with multiple endocrine neoplasia type 1 and related disorders. Am J Hum Genet 1998;63:455–467.
14 Wautot V, Vercherat C, Lespinasse J, et al: Germline mutation profile of MEN1 in multiple endocrine neoplasia type 1: search for correlation between phenotype and the functional domains of the MEN1 protein. Hum Mutat 2002;20: 35–47.
15 Thompson GB, Young WF: Multiple endocrine neoplasia type 1; in Clark O, Duh Q-Y, Kebebew E (eds): Multiple Endocrine Neoplasia Type 1. Philadelphia, Elsevier Saunders, 2005, pp 673–690.
16 Hebert SC: Therapeutic use of calcimimetics. Annu Rev Med 2006;57:349–364.
17 Falchetti A, Cilotti A, Vaggelli L, et al: A patient with MEN1-associated hyperparathyroidism, responsive to cinacalcet. Nat Clin Pract Endocrinol Metab 2008;4: 351–357.
18 Faggiano A, Tavares LB, Tauchmanova L, et al: Effect of treatment with depot somatostatin analogue octreotide on primary hyperparathyroidism (PHP) in multiple endocrine neoplasia type 1 (MEN1) patients. Clin Endocrinol (Oxf) 2008;69:756–762.
19 Eng C: Common alleles of predisposition in endocrine neoplasia. Curr Opin Genet Dev 2010;20:1–6.
20 Ponder BA, Ponder MA, Coffey R, et al: Risk estimation and screening in families of patients with medullary thyroid carcinoma. Lancet 1988;i:397–401.
21 Mulligan LM, Kwok JB, Healey CS, et al: Germ-line mutations of the RET proto-oncogene in multiple endocrine neoplasia type 2A. Nature 1993;363:458–460.
22 Marsh DJ, Hahn MA, Howell VM, Gill AJ: Molecular diagnosis of primary hyperparathyroidism in familial cancer syndromes. Expert Opin Med Diagn 2007;1:377–392.
23 Eng C, Clayton D, Schuffenecker I, et al: The relationship between specific RET proto-oncogene mutations and disease phenotype in multiple endocrine neoplasia type 2. International RET mutation consortium analysis. JAMA 1996; 276:1575–1579.
24 Schuffenecker I, Billaud M, Calender A, et al: RET proto-oncogene mutations in French MEN 2A and FMTC families. Hum Mol Genet 1994;3:1939–1943.
25 Wiesner GL, Snow-Bailey K: Multiple endocrine neoplasia type 2. Gene Reviews. Seattle, University of Washington, 2005, pp 1–25.
26 Machens A, Lorenz K, Dralle H: Individualization of lymph node dissection in RET (rearranged during transfection) carriers at risk for medullary thyroid cancer: value of pretherapeutic calcitonin levels. Ann Surg 2009;250: 305–310.
27 Wells SA Jr, Gosnell JE, Gagel RF, et al: Vandetanib for the treatment of patients with locally advanced or metastatic hereditary medullary thyroid cancer. J Clin Oncol 2010;28:767–772.

Deborah J. Marsh, PhD
Hormones and Cancer Group, Kolling Institute of Medical Research
University of Sydney, E25, Royal North Shore Hospital
St. Leonards NSW 2065 (Australia)
Tel. +61 2 99264500, Fax +61 2 99268484, E-Mail deborah.marsh@sydney.edu.au

Alford RL, Sutton VR (eds): Medical Genetics in the Clinical Practice of ORL.
Adv Otorhinolaryngol. Basel, Karger, 2011, vol 70, pp 91–98

Neurofibromatosis Type 2

D. Gareth R. Evans[a] · Simon K.W. Lloyd[b] · Richard T. Ramsden[b]

[a]Medical Genetics Research Group, Regional Genetics Service and National Molecular Genetics Reference Laboratory, Manchester Academic Health Sciences Centre, Central Manchester Universities Foundation Trust, St. Mary's Hospital,
[b]Department of Otolaryngology, Central Manchester NHS Foundation Trust, Manchester Royal Infirmary, and Salford Royal NHS Foundation Trust, Salford, Manchester, UK

Abstract

Neurofibromatosis type 2 (NF2) is an autosomal-dominant inherited tumour predisposition syndrome caused by mutations in the *NF2* gene on chromosome 22. Affected individuals develop schwannomas characteristically affecting both vestibular nerves leading to hearing loss and eventual deafness. Rehabilitation with brain stem implants and in some cases cochlear implants is improving this outcome. Schwannomas also occur on other cranial nerves, on spinal nerve roots and peripheral nerves. Meningiomas and ependymomas are other tumour features. In excess of 50% of patients represent de novo mutations and as many as 33% are mosaic for the underlying disease causing mutation. Truncating mutations (nonsense, frameshift insertions/deletions) are the most frequent germline events and cause the most severe disease, whilst single and multiple exon deletions are common and are usually associated with milder NF2. A strategy for detection of the latter is vital for a sensitive genetic analysis. NF2 represents a difficult management problem with most patients facing substantial morbidity and reduced life expectancy. Surgery remains the focus of current management although watchful waiting and occasionally radiation treatment have a role. We are seeing the advent of tailored drug therapies aimed at the genetic level and these are likely to provide huge improvements for this devastating, life limiting condition.

Epidemiology

NF2 is an autosomal-dominant disease that usually has a 50% risk of transmission from an affected individual to their offspring. This was first confirmed in a large family reported by Gardner and Frazier in 1930. Fifty to sixty percent of patients have no family history and represent de novo mutations in the NF2 gene [1–3]. Individuals who inherit a pathogenic mutation in the *NF2* gene will almost always develop symptoms by 60 years of age [1]. Although the transmission rate is 50% in the second generation and beyond, the risk of transmission in an apparently isolated patient with NF2 is less than 50% due to mosaicism [4]. This is a phenomenon whereby the NF2 mutation is only present in some of the affected individual's cells but not in all cells. There have only been two epidemiological studies of NF2: one in North West England [5–7] and one in Finland [8]. The birth incidence of NF2 is most probably around 1:33,000 individuals [7], with disease prevalence around 1 in 60,000 [7].

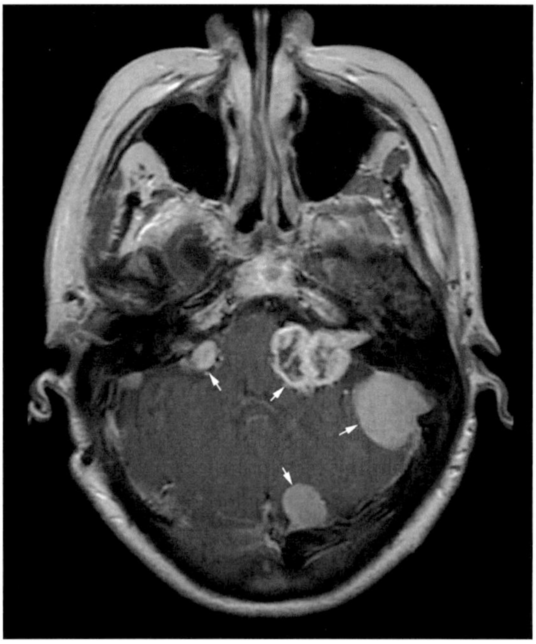

Fig. 1. Cranial MRI showing bilateral VS and meningiomas.

Clinical Description

The first clear description of NF2 was in 1822 by Wishart [9]. Neurofibromatosis type 1 (NF1) was described in 1882 by von Recklinghausen. However, it was Harvey Cushing who described bilateral eighth nerve tumours developing as part of von Recklinghausen disease in 1916 [10]. This description is largely responsible for the confusion between the two conditions which continued for many years.

The hallmark of NF2 is the development of bilateral vestibular schwannomas (VS) (fig. 1). The other main tumour features are schwannomas of the other cranial, spinal and peripheral nerves; meningiomas both intracranial (including optic nerve meningiomas) and intraspinal, and some low-grade central nervous system (CNS) malignancies (ependymomas). Four large clinical studies have now confirmed this clinical picture [1, 11–13]. Although the disease is still classified as 'neurofibromatosis', neurofibromas are relatively infrequent. Individuals may present with cranial meningiomas or a spinal tumour long before the appearance of a VS. There are two forms of the disease. The Wishart type is more aggressive with an onset commonly in the late teens or early twenties. The Gardner type is less aggressive and usually presents in an older age group. Tumours may present very early, particularly cranial meningiomas.

In the same way as sporadic VS, the majority of adults with NF2 present with hearing loss that is usually unilateral at time of onset. Nausea, vomiting or true vertigo are rare symptoms except in late stage disease. A significant proportion of cases (20–30%) present with symptoms from an intracranial meningioma (headaches, seizures), spinal tumour (pain, muscle weakness, paraesthesia), or cutaneous tumour [1, 12–14]. Indeed, the first sign of more severe multi-tumour disease in early childhood is often a non-8th nerve tumour (including a cutaneous tumour), an ocular presentation, or a mononeuropathy which frequently affects the facial nerve [14]. Some children present with a polio-like illness with wasting of muscle groups in a lower limb, which usually does not fully recover. In adulthood, a more generalised symptomtatic severe polyneuropathy occurs in about 3–10% of patients, often associated with an 'onion bulb' appearance on nerve biopsy [1]. Around 40% of patients will show evidence of polyneuropathy on nerve conduction studies [15].

Ophthalmic features are also prominent in NF2. Patients often suffer from reduced visual acuity of various causes. Between 60 and 80% of patients have cataracts and these may present in early life [1, 12, 13]. These can be posterior subcapsular lenticular opacities or cortical wedge opacities. Optic nerve meningiomas can cause visual loss in the first years of life and extensive retinal hamartomas can also affect vision.

The skin is a useful aid to diagnosis, but cutaneous features in NF2 are much more subtle than in NF1. About 70% of NF2 patients have skin related tumours, but only 10% have more than ten skin tumours. The most frequent type is a plaque-like lesion, which is intra-cutaneous, slightly raised and more pigmented than surrounding skin, often with excess hair. More deep-seated subcutaneous nodular tumours can often be felt, sometimes on major peripheral nerves.

Genetics

NF1 and NF2 were eventually recognised as separate genetic and clinical diseases with the localisation of the respective genes to chromosome 17 and 22 [16, 17]. This was followed by the formal clinical delineation at a National Institutes of Health (NIH) consensus meeting in the USA in 1987 [19].

The *NF2* gene was isolated by the simultaneous discovery of constitutional and tumour deletions in a gene coding for a cell membrane-related protein, which has been termed merlin or schwannomin by the two groups who isolated it [2, 3]. This protein is involved in the interaction between actin within the cell cytoskeleton and the cell membrane and appears to suppress tumorigenesis through contact-mediated growth inhibition.

Standard mutation techniques, such as single strand conformational polymorphism (SSCP) analysis or denaturing gradient gel electrophoresis (DGGE), detect between 35% and 66% of pathogenic mutations [21–24]. The majority of these mutations are truncating mutations, leading to a smaller and probably non-functional protein product. Early studies suggested that missense mutations (which result in a complete protein product) and large deletions (which result in no protein product) both cause mild phenotypes. Larger studies of detailed genotype/phenotype correlations in multiple families have confirmed this finding [21–26]. The phenotype is more variable in patients with splice-site mutations, with milder disease in patients with mutations in exons 9–15 [26, 27]. This variation in disease severity is reflected in longer survival for those patients with a missense mutation compared to those with a truncating mutation [26]. Large scale genomic rearrangements may also occur and account for around 15% of NF2 germline aberrations [28, 29]. The sensitivity of genetic testing using sequence analysis and MLPA is around 92% as this is the detection rate in the second generation of NF2 families [30].

A considerable proportion of NF2 patients, particularly milder cases, have mosaic disease, in which only a proportion of cells contain the mutated *NF2* gene. The initiating mutation occurs after conception, leading to two separate cell lineages. The proportion of cells affected depends on how early in development the mutation occurs. Recent evidence suggests that between 20 and 33% of NF2 cases without a family history of the disease are mosaic, mostly carrying the mutation in too small a proportion or none of their lymphocytes to be detected from a blood sample [4, 30–32]. This accounts for the milder disease course in many individuals with unfound mutations, and since only a subset of germ cells (or none) will carry the mutation, there is less than a 50% risk of transmitting the disease to their offspring. However, if an offspring has inherited the mutation, they will have a typical phenotype and usually be more severely affected than their parent, since the offspring will carry the mutation in all of their cells. The mosaic mutation can be detected by analysing tumour material from an affected individual. If an identical mutation is found in two tumours from that individual, this confirms that this is the underlying mosaic mutation even if it cannot be identified in lymphocyte DNA. Their offspring can be tested for the presence of the mutation to exclude NF2. Offspring can also be tested for NF2 if both abnormalities are identified in a single tumour to exclude the disease.

Table 1. Diagnostic criteria for NF2 (these include the NIH criteria with additional criteria)

Bilateral vestibular schwannomas *or* family history of NF2 *plus*
(1) Unilateral VS *or*
(2) Any two of: meningioma, glioma, neurofibroma, schwannoma, posterior subcapsular lenticular opacities
Additional criteria: Unilateral VS *plus* any two of: meningioma, glioma, neurofibroma, schwannoma, and posterior subcapsular opacities
Or
Multiple meningioma (two or more) *plus* unilateral VS *or* any two of: glioma, neurofibroma, schwannoma, and cataract

Diagnosis

The Manchester (modified NIH) diagnostic criteria for NF2 are shown in table 1. The original NIH criteria have been expanded to include patients with no family history who have multiple schwannomas and/or meningiomas, but who have not yet developed bilateral 8th nerve tumours. Patients who have asymmetric involvement are likely to be mosaic [30, 33]. At very young ages (<18 years) individuals presenting with an apparently isolated meningioma [15] or vestibular schwannoma [34] have a 20 and 10% likelihood respectively of developing NF2. However, after 20 years of age this rate drops dramatically and the diagnosis becomes very unlikely after 30 years of age [34].

Differential Diagnosis

The main differential diagnosis of NF2 is schwannomatosis although some patients with multiple non-cranial schwannomas turn out to have mosaic NF2 [30]. Patients fulfilling the most sensitive Manchester criteria are unlikely to be misclassified [35].

Screening Protocol
Children of affected patients should be considered to be at 50% risk of NF2 and screening for NF2 can start at birth with a search for cataracts. Formal screening for VS should start at ten years, as it is rare for tumours to become symptomatic before that time even in severely affected families. Magnetic resonance imaging (MRI) of the head and spine is the mainstay of current screening although annual audiological tests including auditory brainstem response are still a useful adjunct to MRI [36]. VS growth is faster in younger patients, so for asymptomatic at-risk individuals without tumours, MRI screening every 2 years for those younger than 20 years old is recommended. For those older than 20 years MRI screening every 3–5 years should be sufficient. The initial MRI scan could be at around 12 years of age, or 10 years of age in severely affected families. Once tumours are present, MRI screening should probably be at least annual. Spinal tumours are seen in 60–80% of NF2 patients on MRI [37]. Nonetheless, only 25–30% of patients with spinal tumours require a spinal operation from a symptomatic tumour. Spinal MRI only every 3 years is probably sufficient unless there are new symptoms [38]. If no tumours are present on the initial scan a further scan five to ten years later may be reasonable.

In most families it is now possible to develop a genetic test so that screening can be targeted to affected individuals only. Identifying the affected patient's mutation not only allows testing of at risk relatives, but may also give important indicators as to the patient's own prognosis. As 20–33% of de novo NF2 patients are mosaic frozen tumour should be taken at operation (with patient consent) for genetic tests.

NF2 Management

Surgery

VS surgery in NF2 presents unique technical and decision-making challenges. Cerebello-pontine angle CPA schwannomas may have multicentric components from the eighth nerve as well as from adjacent cranial nerves – facial, trigeminal and the lower nerves. As a result the facial nerve may pass though the middle of the tumour mass and be difficult to identify. The principle of surgery is to limit the burden of neurological deficit as far as is possible. Facial nerve preservation is very important in the presence of bilateral disease. Facial paralysis threatens the health of the eye by loss of blink and lacrymation, and if combined with trigeminal damage is a serious threat to vision. Risk is minimised leaving fragments of VS on the facial nerve and if possible by not removing a coexistent facial schwannoma. The patient should be considered holistically. If the vision in the opposite side is poor (not an infrequent occurence in NF2), then surgery should be very conservative. Similar arguments apply to the management of the lower cranial nerves to avoid the problems of bilateral bulbar palsy. In general terms a tumour should not be removed just because it is there. Usually, a VS with good hearing will be treated conservatively until there is a neurosurgical need to remove it. There are occasions, however, when early removal of small tumours will be advised if it is felt possible to preserve hearing or at worst the cochlear nerve for subsequent cochlear implantation. Surgical results are certainly far better when managed by an experienced team [38, 39]. There is clear evidence of a reduction in mortality with a significantly increased life expectancy for NF2 patients managed at three specialty centres in the UK (OR 0.34) [40].

Radiotherapy

The use of radiotherapy is controversial in patients with NF2 although it may be useful in some situations. The same tumour considerations of VS with often multifocal disease make treatment results worse in NF2 than in sporadic disease [41]. It has a role in patients who have particularly aggressive tumours, who are poor surgical candidates or who refuse surgery. This should be weighed against control rates of only 50% compared to a control rate in sporadic VS of 95% [42, 43]. In addition, there is a greater risk of malignant change in NF2 patients compared to sporadic VS [44, 45]. Forty percent of patients retain pre-treatment hearing for at least 3 years. The upper limit of size for radiotherapy is generally a maximum intracranial diameter of 3 cm [42]. It is important to be able to offer both radiotherapy and surgery and both options should be discussed in a balanced fashion. Surgeons should use clinical judgement as to when to recommend radiation therapy [38, 43].

Hearing Rehabilitation

Hearing preservation surgery in patients with NF2 is extremely difficult. Patients often become bilaterally profoundly deaf as a result of the disease or treatment of the disease. Teams experienced in the positioning of brainstem implants can offer partial auditory rehabilitation to those who are deaf, although results are still behind those achievable for cochlear implants. In a few patients, it may be possible to rehabilitate hearing successfully with a cochlear implant if the cochlear nerve is left intact after surgery. However, this is not always possible even in the presence of an intact nerve as its blood supply may be damaged. The Auditory Brainstem Implant (ABI, Cochlear Nucleus Implant) has allowed most recipients to appreciate environmental noise and to enhance their lip reading skills. A small number are able to achieve good open set sentence scores, but as yet the factors that predict outcome are not fully understood.

New Therapies
The NF2 protein appears to impact on multiple intracellular signaling pathways. These pathways include the PI3-kinase, mTOR, Akt, and Raf/MEK/ERK pathways [46].

The progress being made in cellular research especially with regard to pathways in which the NF2 gene product interacts raises the hopes of targeted therapy. Targeting the ERK1, AKT, integrin/focal adhesion kinase/Src/Ras signaling cascades, PDGFRbeta, phosphatidylinositol 3-kinase/protein kinase C/Src/c-Raf pathway,VEG-F and other pathways [46] means that drugs such as bevacizumab [47], elotinib, lapatinib and sorafenib [48] may well bear fruit. Indeed a recent report on 10 patients showed objective radiological improvement in eight VS with bevacizumab [47].

Managing Affected Children
NF2 is being recognised more and more frequently in childhood often before VS have developed. Recognition of the more severe disease course with early presentation and the more atypical features such as mononeuropathy are important [14]. Children often have faster growing tumours and presentation in childhood implies a poorer prognosis [40].

Multidisciplinary Management

NF2 patients should ideally be managed by a multidisciplinary team including a physician (neurologist/geneticist), neurosurgeon, otolaryngologist and neuroradiologist [38]. The complexity of management including potential for therapy means that input from oncologists, paediatricians, ophthalmologists, etc., are likely also to be needed.

Conclusions

NF2 continues to be a condition with considerable morbidity and increased mortality. Multidisciplinary management with early diagnosis is vital for management [38]. Hopefully, new targeted therapies will revolutionise the outcomes in this condition.

References

1 Evans DGR, Huson S, Donnai D, Neary W, Blair V, Newton V, Harris R: A clinical study of type 2 neurofibromatosis. Q J Med 1992;84:603–618.

2 Rouleau GA, Merel P, Lutchman M, Sanson M, Zucman J, Marineau C, Hoang-xuan K, Demczuk S, Desmaze C, Plougastel B, Pulst SM, Lenoir G, Bijlsma E, Fashold R, Dumanski J, de Jong P, Parry D, Eldridge R, Aurias A, Delattre O, Thomas G: Alteration in a new gene encoding a putative membrane-organizing protein causes neuro-fibromatosis type 2. Nature 1993; 363:515–521.

3 Troffater JA, MacCollin MM, Rutter JL, Murrell JR, Duyao MP, Eldridge R, Kley N, Menon AG, Pulaski K, Haase VH, Ambrose CM, Munroe D, Bove C, Haines JL, Martuza RL, MacDonald ME, Seizinger BR, Short PM, Buckler AJ, Gusella JF: A novel moesin-, ezrin-, radixin-like gene is a candidate for the neurofibromatosis 2 tumor suppressor. Cell 1993;72:791–800.

4 Evans DGR, Wallace A, Trueman L, Strachan T: Mosaicism in classical neurofibromatosis type 2: a common mechanism for sporadic disease in tumor prone syndromes? Am J Hum Genet 1998;63:727–736.

5 Evans DGR, Huson SM, Donnai D, Neary W, Blair V, Teare D, Ramsden RT, Harris R: A genetic study of type 2 neurofibromatosis in the north west of England and the UK. I. Prevalence, mutation rate, fitness and confirmation of maternal transmission effect on severity. J Med Genet 1992;29:841–846.

6 Evans DGR, Moran A, King A, Saeed S, Gurusinghe N, Ramsden R: Incidence of vestibular schwannoma and neurofibromatosis 2 in the north west of England over a 10 year period: higher incidence than previously thought. Otol Neurotol 2005;26:93–97.

7 Evans DG, Howard E, Giblin C, Clancy T, Spencer H, Huson SM, Lalloo F: Birth incidence and prevalence of tumour prone syndromes: estimates from a UK genetic family register service. Am J Med Genet 2010;152A:327–332.
8 Antinheimo J, Sankila R, Carpén O, Pukkala E, Sainio M, Jääskeläinen J: Population-based analysis of sporadic and type 2 neurofibromatosis-associated meningiomas and schwannomas. Neurology 2000;54:71–76.
9 Wishart JH: Case of tumours in the skull, dura mater, and brain. Edinburgh Med Surg J 1822;18:393–397.
10 Cushing H: Tumors of the Nervus Acusticus and the Syndrome of the Cerebello-Pontine Angle. Saunders, Philadelphia, 1917.
11 Kanter WR, Eldridge R, Fabricant R, Allen JC, Koerber T: Central neurofibromatosis with bilateral acoustic neuroma: genetic, clinical and biochemical distinctions from peripheral neurofibromatosis. Neurol 1980;30:851–859.
12 Parry DM, Eldridge R, Kaiser-Kupfer MI, Bouzas EA, Pikus A, Patronas N: Neurofibromatosis 2 (NF2): clinical characteristics of 63 affected individuals and clinical evidence for heterogeneity. Am J Med Genet 1994;52:450–451.
13 Mautner VF, Lindenau M, Baser ME, et al: The neuroimaging and clinical spectrum of neurofibromatosis 2. Neurosurgery 1996;38:880–885.
14 Evans DGR, Ramsden R, Birch J: Paediatric presentation of type 2 neurofibromatosis. Arch Dis Child 1999; 81:496–499.
15 Sperfeld AD, Hein C, Schroder JM, Ludolph AC, Hanemann CO: Occurrence and characterization of peripheral nerve involvement in neurofibromatosis type 2. Brain 2002;125:996–1004.
16 Seizinger BR, Rouleau GA, Ozelius LG, Ozelius LJ, Faryniarz AG, Iannazzi J, Hobbs W, Roy JC, Falcone B, Huson S: Genetic linkage of von Recklinghausen neurofibromatosis to the nerve growth factor receptor gene. Cell 1987;49:589–594.
17 Rouleau G, Seizinger BR, Ozelius LG, Hobbs WJ, Trofatter JA, Seizinger BR, Martuza RL, Superneau DW, Conneally PM, Gusella JF: Genetic linkage analysis of bilateral acoustic neurofibromatosis to a DNA marker on chromosome 22. Nature 1987;329:246–248
18 National Institutes of Health Consensus Development Conference Statement on Neurofibromatosis. Arch Neurol 1987; 45:575–579.
19 Seizinger BR, Martuza RL, Gusella JF: Loss of genes on chromosome 22 in tumorigenesis of human acoustic neuroma. Nature 1986;322:644–647.
20 MacCollin M, Ramesh V, Jacoby LB, Louis DN, Rubio MP, Pulaski K, Trofatter JA, Short MP, Bove C, Eldridge R: Mutational analysis of patients with neurofibromatosis 2. Am J Hum Genet 1994; 55:314–320.
21 Parry DM, MacCollin M, Kaiser-Kupfer MI, Pulaski K, Nicholson HS, Boleseta M, Eldridge R, Gusella JF: Germ-line mutations in the neurofibromatosis 2 gene: correlations with disease severity and retinal abnormalities. Am J Hum Genet 1996;59:529–539.
22 Ruttledge MH, Andermann AA, Phelan CM, Claudio JO, Han F-Y, Chretien N, Rangaratnam S, MacCollin M, Short P, Parry D, Michels V, Riccardi VM, Weksberg R, Kitamura K, Bradburn JM, Hall BD, Propping P, Rouleau GA: Type of mutation in the neurofibromatosis type 2 gene (NF2) frequently determines severity of disease. Am J Hum Genet 1996;59:331–342.
23 Kluwe L, Bayer S, Baser ME, Hazim W, Haase W, Funsterer C, Mautner VF: Identification of NF2 germ-line mutations and comparison with neurofibromatosis 2 phenotypes [published erratum in Hum Genet 1997;99(2):292]. Hum Genet 1996;98:534–538.
24 Kluwe L, MacCollin M, Tatagiba M, Thomas S, Hazim W, Haase W, Mautner VF: Phenotypic variability associated with 14 splice-site mutations in the NF2 gene. Am J Med Genet 1998;77:228–233.
25 Evans DGR, Trueman L, Wallace A, Mason S, Strachan T: Genotype/phenotype correlations in type 2 neurofibromatosis: evidence for more severe disease with truncating mutations. J Med Genet 1998;35:450–455.
26 Baser ME, Kuramoto L, Joe H, Kuramoto L, Joe H, Friedman JM, Wallace AJ, Ramsden RT, Evans DG: Genotype-phenotype correlations for nervous system tumors in neurofibromatosis. 2. A population-based study. Am J Hum Genet 2004;75:231–239.
27 Baser ME, Kuramoto L, Woods RH, Friedman JM, Wallace AJ, Ramsden RT, Olschwang S, Bijlsma E, Kalamarides M, Papi L, Kato L, Evans DG: The location of constitutional neurofibromatosis 2 (NF2) splice-site mutations is associated with the severity of NF2. J Med Genet 2005;42:540–546.
28 Tsilchorozidou T, Menko, F, Lalloo F, Kidd A, Da Silva R, Smith P, Malcolmson A, Dore J, Madan K, Brown A, Yovos JG, Tsaligopoulos M, Vogiatzis N, Wallace A, Evans DGR: Constitutional rearrangements of chromosome 22 as a cause of neurofibromatosis type 2. J Med Genet 2004;41:529–534.
29 Kluwe L, Nygren AO, Errami A, Heinrich B, Matthies C, Tatagiba M, Mautner V: Screening for large mutations of the NF2 gene. Genes Chromosomes Cancer 2005; 42:384–391.
30 Evans DGR, Ramsden RT, Shenton A, Gokhale C, Bowers NL, Huson SM, Wallace A: Mosaicism in NF2 an update of risk based on uni/bilaterality of vestibular schwannoma at presentation and sensitive mutation analysis including MLPA. J Med Genet 2007;44:424–428.
31 Kluwe L, Mautner VF, Heinrich B, Dezube R, Jacoby LB, Friedrich RE, MacCollin M: Molecular study of frequency of mosaicism in neurofibromatosis 2 patients with bilateral vestibular schwannomas. J Med Genet 2003; 40:109–114.
32 Moyhuddin A, Baser ME, Watson C, Purcell S, Ramsden RT, Heiberg A, Wallace AJ, Evans DGR: Somatic mosaicism in neurofibromatosis 2: prevalence and risk of disease transmission to offspring. J Med Genet 2003;40:459–463.
33 Evans DGR, Ramsden RT, Shenton A, Gokhale C, Bowers NL, Huson SM, Wallace A: What are the implications in individuals with unilateral vestibular schwannoma and other neurogenic tumors? J Neurosurg 2008;108:92–96.
34 Evans DGR, Ramsden RT, Shenton A, Gokhale C, Bowers NL, Huson SM, Wallace A: Should NF2 mutation screening be undertaken in patients with an apparently isolated vestibular schwannoma? Clin Genet 2007;71:354–358.
35 Baser ME, Friedman JM, Wallace AJ, Ramsden RT, Joe H, Evans DGR: Evaluation of diagnostic criteria for neurofibromatosis 2. Neurology 2002; 59:1759–1765.

36 Evans DGR, Newton V, Neary W, Baser ME, Wallace A, MacLeod R, Jenkins JPR, Gillespie J, Ramsden R: Use of MRI and audiological tests in pre-symptomatic diagnosis of type 2 neurofibromatosis (NF2). J Med Genet 2000;37:944–947.
37 King A, Biggs N, Ramsden RT, Wallace A, Gillespie J, Evans DGR: Spinal tumors in neurofibromatosis type 2: is emerging knowledge of genotype predictive of natural history? J Neurosurg Spine 2005; 2:574–579.
38 Evans DGR, Baser ME, O'Reilly B, Rowe J, Gleeson M, Saeed S, King A, Huson S, Kerr R, Thomas N, Irving R, MacFarlane R, Ferner R, McLeod R, Moffat D, Ramsden R: Management of the patient and family with neurofibromatosis 2: a consensus conference statement. Br J Neurosurg 2005;19:5–12.
39 Slattery WH, Brackmann DE, Hitselberger W. Hearing preservation in neurofibromatosis type 2. Am J Otol 1998; 19:638–643.
40 Baser ME, Friedman JM, Aeschilman D, Joe H, Wallace AJ, Ramsden RT, Evans DGR: Predictors of the risk of mortality in neurofibromatosis 2. Am J Hum Genet 2002;71:715–723.
41 Sobel RA, Wang Y: Vestibular (acoustic) schwannomas: histological features in neurofibromatosis 2 and in unilateral cases. J Neuropathol Exp Neurol 1993; 52:106–113.
42 Rowe JG, Radatz M, Walton L, Kemeny AA: Stereotactic radiosurgery for type 2 neurofibromatosis acoustic neuromas: patient selection and tumour size. Stereotact Funct Neurosurg 2002; 79:107–116.
43 Rowe JG, Radatz MW, Walton L, Soanes T, Rodgers J, Kemeny AA: Clinical experience with gamma knife stereotactic radiosurgery in the management of vestibular schwannomas secondary to type 2 neurofibromatosis. J Neurol Neurosurg Psychiatry 2003;74:1288–1293.
44 Baser ME, Evans DGR, Jackler RK, Sujansky E, Rubenstein A: Malignant peripheral nerve sheath tumors, radiotherapy, and neurofibromatosis 2. Br J Cancer 2000;82:998.
45 Evans DGR, Birch JM, Ramsden RT, Sharif S, Baser ME: Malignant transformation and new primary tumours after therapeutic radiation for benign disease: substantial risks in certain tumour-prone syndromes. J Med Genet 2006;43: 289–294.
46 Evans DG, Kalamarides M, Hunter-Schaedle K, et al: Consensus recommendations to accelerate clinical trials for neurofibromatosis type 2. Clin Cancer Res 2009;15:5032–5039.
47 Plotkin SR, Stemmer-Rachamimov AO, Barker FG 2nd, Halpin C, Padera TP, Tyrrell A, Sorensen AG, Jain RK, di Tomaso E: Hearing improvement after bevacizumab in patients with neurofibromatosis type 2. N Engl J Med 2009; 361:358–367.
48 Hanemann CO: Magic but treatable? Tumours due to loss of merlin. Brain 2008;131:606–615.

Prof. D. Gareth R. Evans
Genetic Medicine, St. Mary's Hospital
Oxford Road
Manchester M13 9WL (UK)
Tel. +44 161 276 6228, Fax +44 161 276 6145, E-Mail gareth.evans@cmft.nhs.uk

Alford RL, Sutton VR (eds): Medical Genetics in the Clinical Practice of ORL.
Adv Otorhinolaryngol. Basel, Karger, 2011, vol 70, pp 99–106

Hereditary Paragangliomas

Margarita Raygada[a] · Barbara Pasini[c] · Constantine A. Stratakis[b]

[a]Section on Clinical Genomics, Program Reproductive and Adult Endocrinology and [b]Section on Endocrinology and Genetics, Program on Developmental Endocrinology and Genetics, Eunice Kennedy Shriver National Institute of Child Health and Human Development, National Institutes of Health, Bethesda, Md., USA; [c]Department of Genetics, Biology and Biochemistry, University of Turin, Turin, Italy

Abstract

Paragangliomas (PGL) and pheochromocytomas (PCC) are rare, usually benign tumors that originate from the neuroendocrine tissue along the paravertebral axis. Up to 35% of these tumors may be hereditary; they are associated with germline mutations in genes encoding subunits of the succinate dehydrogenase (SDH) enzyme complex in the context of the familial PGL syndromes, PGL1, 3 and 4 caused by mutations in the *SDHD*, *SDHC* and *SDHB* genes, respectively. Another familial PGL syndrome, PGL2, is caused by mutations in *SDHAF2/SDH5*, which encodes for a molecule that is an accessory to the function of the SDH enzyme and its SDHA subunit. Less frequently, mutations in the genes responsible for Von Hippel Lindau disease (VHL), multiple endocrine neoplasia type 2 (MEN2), and neurofibromatosis type 1 (NF1) are also found in patients with hereditary PGL and PCC. Recently mutations were found in the *SDHA* subunit in a limited number of patients with PGL and/or PCC. The *SDHB*, *SDHC* and *SDHD* gene mutations (but not *SDHA*) can also be found in patients with PGL and/or PCC and gastrointestinal stromal tumors (GISTs), also known as the Carney-Stratakis syndrome; *SDHB* mutations, in particular, may also predispose to thyroid and renal cancer, and possibly other tumors. A new gene was recently found to predispose to PGL and/or PCC when mutated is TMEM127. In this text, we provide an overview of the genetics of PGLs and related conditions with an emphasis on genetic risk assessment, prevention, and prognosis.

Historically, paragangliomas were thought of as benign tumors derived from specialized periocytes in the glomus complexes [1]; we now know that they originate from the chromaffin-negative glomus cells of the embryonic neural crest. These cells which migrated in close association with the autonomic nervous system ganglia are dispersed from the middle ear and the skull to the pelvic floor. Based on their anatomical distribution, and autonomic function, PGLs can be divided into two categories: (1) extra-adrenal tumors of the head and neck (HNPGLs) usually located at the carotid bifurcation, along the vagal nerve, in the jugular foramen, or in the middle ear space, and (2) tumors located below the neck which are most commonly found in the adrenal medulla (pheochromocytoma; PCC), urinary bladder, and the upper mediastinum. The incidence of clinically significant PGLs in the general population is approximately 1:30,000 to 1:100,000; in most cases, there is high morbidity but mortality remains low; early screening for familial cases and intervention are essential for good prognosis.

All types of PGLs and PCCs can occur in both sporadic and hereditary forms; approximately 7–10 to 50% of cases of PGLs are familial or present as bilateral or multiple primary tumors thus suggesting a genetic predisposition [2–5]; the proportion of PGLs due to an inherited predisposition is close to 35% [6]. Hereditary syndromes associated with PGLs include Von Hippel Lindau disease (VHL), multiple endocrine neoplasia type 2 (MEN2), and neurofibromatosis type 1 (NF1) and the PGL syndromes (PGLs 1–4) and Carney-Stratakis syndrome or dyad. In NF1, adrenal PCCs occur in nearly 1% of patients [7, 8].

In general, extra-adrenal PGLs are associated with a greater risk of metastasis (23.9%) than adrenal PCCs (6.7%) [9–11]. Recent studies have identified an additional locus on chromosome 1p36 that also seems to predispose to PCCs (gene *KIF1Bβ*) [12, 13]. In 2000, mutations in the succinate dehyrogenase subunit D *(SDHD)* gene were found to be associated with hereditary PGLs [14]; this finding was followed by more mutations in SDH subunit genes that are also associated with hereditary PGLs. These are: three loci on chromosome 11 and 1, named PGL1 on 11q23 [15–18], PGL2 on 11q13.1 [19, 20] and PGL3 on 1q21–23 [21, 22]. Co-occurrence of both PGLs and PCCs is well documented in these syndromes [23]. *SDHD* (OMIM 602690) is responsible for PGL1 in familial PGLs [14], whereas two other subunits of this mitochondrial enzyme, *SDHC* (PGL3, OMIM 602413) and *SDHB* (PGL4, 1p36, OMIM 185470) are also associated with heritable PCC and/or PGL [24, 25]. The gene responsible for PGL2 was recently identified to be *SDHAF2* (also known as *SDH5*), encoding a protein necessary for flavination of the A subunit of the SDH enzyme, SDHA (PGL2, 11q13.1, OMIM 601650) [26].

The genetic predisposition to HNPGLs and adrenal/extra-adrenal PGLs caused by heterozygous mutations by SDHD, SDHC, and SDHB is transmitted in an autosomal dominant fashion with age-dependent and incomplete penetrance [24, 25]. Mutations in the *SDHD* gene show a parent-of-origin effect (transmitted mostly from the father) [4, 15]. Despite this pattern of inheritance, *SDHD* shows bi-allelic expression in normal tissues and neural crest derived cancers with no promoter hyper-methylation in neuroendocrine tissues and related tumours [27]. In 2009, Hao et al. [26] evaluated a previously reported large Dutch family with an autosomal-dominant pattern of PGLs; they identified a mutation (G-to-A transition at nucleotide 232 of exon 2) in the *SDHAF2* gene [26]. The pattern of inheritance seen in this family was suggestive of an SDHD-like inheritance. However, more studies are needed to elucidate the mechanism. More recently, mutations in SDHA were reported in a limited number of kindreds with PGL and/or PCC (see below).

Herited Predisposition to Paragangliomas: Epidemiology and Risk Assessment

In a recent report, we reviewed 95 studies of *SDH* germline mutations (57 in *SDHD*, 54 in *SDHB* and 13 in *SDHC*) in patients affected by tumours related to the 'PGL/PCC syndromes' [29]. This review included all published reports cited in the LOVD *SDH* gene databases by July 2008. For the purpose of the current chapter, we will focus primarily on epidemiology, management, risk assessment, and preventive measures.

Prevalence and Clinical Manifestations of PGL Syndromes

PGL syndromes involve either sympathetic paraganglia (mainly abdominal, adrenal or extra-adrenal) or parasympathetic organs in the head and neck region (mainly carotid bifurcation, the jugular bulb (the tympanic plexus on the promontory or the vagal nerve). Table 1 provides a summary of the prevalence of *SDHB*, *SDHD*, and *SDHC* mutations in sporadic cases of PGL, and table 2 provides a summary of SDHB, SDHC, and SDHD mutations in malignant tumors PGL-PCC. Sixty-one percent of *SDHD*-mutated index cases have a positive family history, while 69% of

Table 1. SDH germline mutations in series of sporadic or unselected patients with adrenal (PHEO) or extra-adrenal (PGL) pheochromocytoma

Tumor type	Number of cases	SDHB	SDHC	SDHD	References (population)
Sporadic PHEO-PGL	24	2 (8.3%)	0	0	Astuti et al., 2001 (English)
Sporadic PHEO-PGL 14 adrenal, 4 extra-adrenal	18	n.d.	n.d.	2 (11.1%)	Gimm et al., 2000 (German)
Sporadic PHEO-PGL	271	12 (4.4%)	n.d.	11 (4%)	Neumann et al., 2002 (German, Polish)
Adrenal	241	6 (2.5%)		7 (2.9%)	
Extra-adrenal	30	6 (20%)		4 (13.3%)	
Multiple tumours	26	0 (0%)		4 (15.4%)	
Sporadic PHEO-PGL	304	16 (5.3%)	neg	13 (4.3%)	Neumann et al., 2004 (German, Polish)
Sporadic PHEO-PGL	371	21 (5.7%)	0	21 (5.7%)	Schiavi et al., 2005 (German, Polish and other countries)
Sporadic PHEO-PGL including multiple tumors	947	59 (6.2%)	neg	25 (2.6%)	Erlic et al., 2009 (European-American)
Sporadic PHEO-PGL	84	8 (9.5%)	n.d.	0	Gimenez-Roqueplo et al., 2003 (French)
Adrenal	69	3 (4.3%)			
Adrenal benign	57	1 (1.7%)			
Adrenal malignant	12	2 (16.7)			
Extra-adrenal	15	5 (33.3%)			
Sporadic PHEO-PGL	258	18 (7%)	0	3 (1.2%)	Amar et al., 2005 (French)
Sporadic PGL >35 years, benign	40	6 (15%)	0	0	Burnichon et al., 2009 (French)
Sporadic PHEO-PGL	213	1/47 (2%)	n.d.	2/126 (1.6%)	Korpershoek et al., 2006 (Dutch)
Sporadic PHEO-PGL	18	0	0	0	Persu et al., 2008 (Belgian)
PHEO collected anonymously	35	1 (2.8%)	n.d.	2 (5.7%)	Cascòn et al., 2004 (Spanish)
Sporadic PHEO-PGL single tumors	119	12 (10%)	0	3 (2.2%)	Cascòn et al., 2009 (Spanish)
Adrenal	95	2 (2.1%)	0	0	
Extra-adrenal	24	10 (41.6%)	0	1 (4.2%)	

Data on the prevalence of *SDH* germline mutations in sporadic non-syndromic PHEOs/PGLs have been derived from 13 studies in which the family history was clearly indicated. n.d. = Analysis not done.

Table 2. SDH germline mutations in series of malignant adrenal (PHEO) or extra-adrenal (PGL) pheochromocytoma

Tumor type	Number of cases	SDHB	SDHC	SDHD	References (population)
Malignant PHEO-PGL	44	13–18 (30–41%)	n.d.	n.d.	Brouwers et al., 2006 (NIH – USA) 5 cases with genetic variants
Adrenal	13	2 (15.4%)			
Extra-adrenal	29	16 (55.2%)			
Uncertain	2	0 (0%)			
Malignant PHEO-PGL	9	1 (11%)	n.d.	0	Isobe et al., 2007 (Japanese)
Adrenal	5	0			
Extra-adrenal	4	1 (25%)			
Malignant PHEO-PGL	28	6–7 (21–25%)	n.d.	1–2 (3.6–7%)	Klein et al., 2008 (USA) 2 cases with genetic variants
Adrenal	12	0		2 (16.7%)	
Extra-adrenal	16	7 (43.8)		0	
Malignant PHEO-PGL	88	20 (22.7%)	n.d.	1 (1.1%)	Erlic et al., 2009 (European-American)
Malignant PHEO-PGL	54	23 (42.6%)	n.d.	0	Amar et al., 2007 (French)
Syndromic	5	2 (40%)			
Sporadic	49	21 (42.8%)			
Adrenal	29	7 (24.1%)			
Extra-adrenal	25	16 (64%)			
Malignant PGL-HNPGL	49	36 (73.5%)	0 (0%)	4 (8.2%)	Burnichon et al., 2009 (French)
Thoracic, abdominal, pelvis	24	20 (83.3%)	0 (0%)	1 (4.1%)	
HNPGL	11	6 (54.5%)	0 (0%)	0 (0%)	
Multiple tumors	14	10 (71.4%)	0 (0%)	3 (21.4%)	
Malignant HNPGL	33	13 (39.4%)	0 (0%)	9 (27.3%)	Neumann et al., 2009 (55% German, 45% other countries)
Total malignant PHEO/PGLs	305	112/305 (36.7%)		15/261 (5.7%)	combined data

Data on the prevalence of *SDH* germline mutations among malignant PHEOs/PGLs have been derived from 7 studies giving a general frequency of 42.4% with a marked predominance of *SDHB* mutations. In two studies, together with deleterious mutations, n.d. = Analysis not done.

SDHB mutations carriers have an apparent negative family history. The few *SDHC* mutated cases described to date have a positive family history in 62.5% of the cases. Therefore, the prevalence of *SDHB* germline mutations among sporadic cases is somewhat higher than that one of *SDHD*. Very few sporadic cases have been reported with *SDHC* germline mutations (0.6%). The prevalence of *SDHAF2*/*SDH5* mutations has not been well described to date; only one study has been reported so far [26, 28]. In summary, the prevalence of *SDH* mutations is as follows: sporadic extra-adrenal tumours (29.4%), malignant tumours (42.4%, table 2) and pediatric cases (29%) with strong preponderance of *SDHB* mutations in all categories (RET, NF1, VHL, MEN, SDHC, SDHB, SDHD). *SDH* mutations seem less frequent than *RET* and *VHL* in bilateral or familial adrenal PCCs. Higher *SDH* mutations frequencies can be found in cases affected by HNPGLs outside the area of the Low Countries (Belgium, The Netherlands and some adjacent lands). The general prevalence of mutations among sporadic, multiple and familial HNPGLs is 19, 71.4 and 96.3%, respectively, with a strong predominance of *SDHD* germline mutations among multiple (71.4%) and familial cases (68.4%), in accordance to the overall higher penetrance of mutations of this genes.

We also reported on the analysis of the clinical manifestations of 689 published carriers of deleterious mutations in *SDHB* (264), *SDHC* (30) and *SDHD* (395) which led to the recognition of a genotype-phenotype correlation [see 29, for review] confirmed by other recent studies [30, 31]. In summary, median age at diagnosis of the first tumour is similar in *SDHB* and *SDHD* mutations carriers (32 and 33 years of age, respectively) and lower than that in *SDHC* mutation carriers (38 years). Approximately 25% of affected *SDHB* carriers have been diagnosed in the first and second decades of life while only 15% of *SDHD* mutation carriers and no *SDHC* mutation carriers have been diagnosed in the first decade of life. Multiple primary tumours are frequently observed in *SDHD* mutation carriers (79%, 167/211 with available information, 66.9% (87/130) while patients with *SDHB* and *SDHC* mutations have single tumours in 67 and 73% of the cases, respectively [30]. The most frequent phenotype associated with *SDHB* germline mutations is the development of extra-adrenal PGL (53%, 140/264, [30]), mainly abdominal (including pelvis and retro-peritoneum) but also thoracic, mediastinal and cervical. Twenty percent of cases present with adrenal PCC alone or associated with PGL (52/264) and another 20% of cases develop only HNPGL (52/264). On the contrary, *SDHD*-affected carriers presented with only HNPGL, single or multiple, in 78% of cases (305/395[YUN1]) while adrenal PCC and/or extra-adrenal PGL are the sole manifestations in 8% (31/395) and 1% (1/395) of cases. Overall 98% of SDHD affected patients develop a HNPGL during follow-up [30]. Among the 30 *SDHC* affected carriers in our review, 87% (26/30) presented with HNPGL alone (87.5% 14/16) [30] while PGL and PCC occurred more rarely. Finally, the prevalence of multiple tumours among *SDHD* mutation carriers is 30–74 vs. 12–28% in *SDHB* carriers. The risk for malignant tumours in *SDHB* carriers is 34–37.5% (37.5%, 36/96 [30]) versus 0–8% in *SDHD* carriers (3.1%, 4/130 [30]). The risk for malignancy for each type of tumor is based on reported cases; many studies are still analysing data on newer cases and these associated risks may change as more cases are reported. Data about the penetrance of SDH mutations (i.e. the risk of developing a tumor for an asymptomatic carrier) can be derived from three major studies [31–33] dealing with a total of 482 (42 + 82 + 358) SDHB and 128 (35 + 30 + 63) SDHD mutation carriers. *SDHB* mutation carriers have a life time cancer risk of 76 with 50% penetrance by age 35–45 years while *SDHD* carriers who inherited the mutation from their father seem to have a life time cancer risk of 85–100% with penetrance of 50% by age 30–40 years. Considering the tumour location, all studies recognized a higher risk for extra-adrenal paragangliomas in *SDHB* mutation carriers, and a higher risk for HNPGLs in *SDHD* mutation carriers. The lifetime risk of developing a renal tumor is higher in SDHB carriers (14 vs. 8% in SDHD) and mutations in all three genes can be associated with gastrointestinal stromal tumors too.

Management of Patients with PGL

Genetic testing of the different mutations associated with PGLs should be done based on the clinical presentation, medical history, family history, and previous testing of relatives. Guidelines for stepwise testing have been recently published and include a detailed family history, tumor size, location, prior history of surgeries, and clinical presentation [32–36]. However, the efficacy of these approaches in preventing disease has not been validated. The approach for managing and counseling PGL patients should include several one-on-one in-person sessions. These meetings can be divided in two categories:

- Pre-test, to make sure that the person understands the implications of a positive test, and that he or she has enough and balanced information to be able to formulate a truly informed consent.
- Post-test, if the person decides to proceed with testing: description of diagnosis, prognosis, assessment of understanding of current treatment and/or management, explanation of recurrence risk, testing of relatives, future options (including prenatal diagnosis for younger patients), and coping with the results.

These sessions are aimed at exploring the impact of the diagnosis on both affected and unaffected family members, assisting families and individuals as they adjust to the diagnosis, and to always be non-directive. These measures are important because of the uncertainty associated with these mutations and the inability to predict with accuracy the appearance and location of tumors, as well as their tendency to recur. The critical components of this process include ascertainment of medical and family history, determination and communication of risk (including risk of malignancy, assessment of risk perception, education regarding the genetics of PGL syndromes, and discussion of prevention and screening options). The prevention and screening options include urine, blood and imaging tests as indicated by the clinical presentation and the type of tumors. In addition to informed decision-making regarding genetic testing, primary outcomes of genetic counseling for PGL syndromes should include decreased worry, increased sense of control, and improved accuracy of risk perception. If left untreated, PGLs can result in significant clinical morbidity and mortality; early treatment and the identification of at risk individuals are thus imperative. The counseling approach highlighted above is aimed at improving adherence to screening recommendations, and thus decreasing morbidity and mortality.

The clinical manifestations of PGLs are broad and the majority of symptoms can mimic minor ailments (e.g. headaches, palpitations). Therefore, once a mutation has been identified individuals should be monitored closely with a lower threshold for further evaluation of symptoms by a physician. Many studies are on the way that will characterize further the genotype-phenotype correlations, with the hope that more specific guidelines can be generated for this patient population. More recently, mutations in SDHA were reported in a limited number of patients with PGL and/or PCC [37]. Additionally, a new gene was identified that predisposes to non-syndromic PGLs and/or PCC [38, 39]. The impact of these new discoveries in genetic risk counseling is currently unknown.

References

1 Winship T, Kloop CT, Jenkins WH: Glomus Jugularis Tumors. Cancer 1948;1:441.

2 Parry DM, Li FP, Strong LC, Carney JA, Schottenfeld D, Reimer RR, Grufferman S: Carotid body tumors in humans: genetics and epidemiology. J Natl Cancer Inst 1982;68:573–578.

3 Grufferman S, Gillman MW, Pasternak LR, Peterson CL, Young WG Jr: Familial carotid body tumors: case report and epidemiologic review. Cancer 1980;46:2116–2122.

4 van der Mey AG, Maaswinkel-Mooy PD, Cornelisse CJ, Schmidt PH, van de Kamp JJ: Genomic imprinting in hereditary glomus tumours: evidence for new genetic theory. Lancet 1989;ii:1291–1294.

5 Sobol SM, Dailey JC: Familial multiple cervical paragangliomas: report of a kindred and review of the literature. Otolaryngol Head Neck Surg 1990;102: 382–390.

6 Drovdlic CM, Myers EN, Peters JA, Baysal BE, Brackmann DE, Slattery WH 3rd, Rubinstein WS: Proportion of heritable paraganglioma cases and associated clinical characteristics. Laryngoscope 2001;111:1822–1827.

7 Maher ER, Eng C: The pressure rises: update on the genetics of pheochromocytoma. Hum Mol Genet 2002;11:2347–2354.

8 Bausch B, Borozdin W, Mautner VF, European-American Phaeochromocytoma Registry Study Group: Germline NF1 mutational spectra and loss-of-heterozygosity analyses in patients with pheochromocytoma and neurofibromatosis type 1. J Clin Endocrinol Metab 2007;92:2784–2792.

9 Amar L, Servais A, Gimenez-Roquelpo AP, Zinzindohoue F, Chatellier G, Plouin PF: Year of diagnosis, features at presentation, and risk of recurrence in patients with pheochromocytoma or secreting paraganglioma. J Clin Endocrinol Metab 2005;90:2110–2116.

10 Khorram-Manesh A, Ahlman H, Nilsson O, et al: Long term outcome of a large series of patients surgically treated for pheochromocytoma. J Intern Med 2005; 258:55–66.

11 Goldstein RE, O'Neill JA Jr, Holcomb GW 3rd, et al: Clinical experience over 48 years with pheochromocytoma. Ann Sug 1999;229:755–764.

12 Schlisio S, Kenchappa RS, Vredeveld LC, et al: The kinesin KIF1Bbeta acts downstream from EglN3 to induce apoptosis and is a potential 1p36 tumor suppressor. Genes Dev 2008;22:884–893.

13 Yeh IT, Lenci RE, Qin Y, et al: A germline mutation of the KIF1B beta gene on 1p36 in a family with neural and non-neural tumors. Hum Genet 2008;124: 279–285.

14 Baysal BE, Ferrell RE, Willett-Brozick JE, et al: Mutations in SDHD, a mitochondrial complex II gene, in hereditary paraganglioma. Science 2000;287:848–851.

15 Heutink P, van der Mey AG, Sandkuijl LA, et al: A gene subject to genomic imprinting and responsible for hereditary paragangliomas maps to chromosome 11q23-qter. Hum Mol Genet 1992; 1:7–10.

16 Heutink P, van Schothorst EM, van der Mey AG, et al: Further localization of the gene for hereditary paragangliomas and evidence for linkage in unrelated families. Eur J Hum Genet 1994;2: 148–158.

17 Baysal BE, Farr JE, Rubinstein WS, et al. Fine mapping of an imprinted gene for familial nonchromaffin paragangliomas, on chromosome 11q23. Am J Hum Genet 1997;60:121–132.

18 Milunsky J, DeStefano AL, Huang XL, et al: Familial paragangliomas: linkage to chromosome 11q23 and clinical implications. Am J Med Genet 1997;72:66–70.

19 Mariman EC, van Beersum SE, Cremers CW, van Baars FM, Ropers HH: Analysis of a second family with hereditary non-chromaffin paragangliomas locates the underlying gene at the proximal region of chromosome 11q. Hum Genet 1993; 91:357–361.

20 Mariman EC, van Beersum SE, Cremers CW, Struycken PM, Ropers HH: Fine mapping of a putatively imprinted gene for familial non-chromaffin paragangliomas to chromosome 11q13.1: evidence for genetic heterogeneity. Hum Genet 1995;95:56–62.

21 Niemann S, Steinberger D, Müller U: PGL3, a third, not maternally imprinted locus in autosomal dominant paraganglioma. Neurogenetics 1999;2:167–170.

22 Niemann S, Becker-Follmann J, Nürnberg G, et al: Assignment of PGL3 to chromosome 1 (q21–q23) in a family with autosomal dominant non-chromaffin paraganglioma. Am J Med Genet 2001;98:32–36.

23 Sato T, Saito H, Yoshinaga K, Shibota Y, Sasano N: Concurrence of carotid body tumor and pheochromocytoma. Cancer 1974;34:1787–1795.

24 Niemann S, Müller U: Mutations in SDHC cause autosomal dominant paraganglioma, type 3. Nat Genet 2000;26: 268–270.

25 Astuti D, Latif F, Dallol A, et al: Gene mutations in the succinate dehydrogenase subunit SDHB cause susceptibility to familial pheochromocytoma and to familial paraganglioma. Am J Hum Genet 2001;69:49–54.

26 Hao HX, Khalimonchuk O, Schraders M, Dephoure N, Bayley JP, Kunst H, Devilee P, Cremers CW, Schiffman JD, Bentz BG, Gygi SP, Winge DR, Kremer H, Rutter J: SDH5, a gene required for flavination of succinate dehydrogenase, is mutated in paraganglioma. Science 2009;28:1139–1142.

27 Baysal BE, Ferrell RE, Willett-Brozick JE, et al: Mutations in SDHD, a mitochondrial complex II gene, in hereditary paraganglioma. Science 2000;287:848–851.

28 Van Baars, FM, Cremers CWRJ, van den Broek P, Veldman JE: Familial non-chromaffinic paragangliomas (glomus tumors): clinical and genetic aspects. Acta Otolaryng 1981;91:589–593.

29 Pasini B, Stratakis CA: SDH mutations in tumorigenesis and inherited endocrine tumours: lesson from the phaeochromocytoma-paraganglioma syndromes. J Intern Med 2009;266:19–42.

30 Burnichon N, Rohmer V, Amar L, Herman P, et al: PGL.NET network. J Clin Endocrinol Metab 2009;94:2817–2827.

31 Ricketts CJ, Forman JR, Rattenberry E, et al: Tumor risks and genotype-phenotype-proteotype analysis in 358 patients with germline mutations in SDHB and SDHD. Hum Mutat 2010;31:41–51.
32 Neumann HP, Eng C. The approach to the patient with paraganglioma. J Clin Endocrinol Metab 2009;94:2677–2683.
33 Benn DE, Richardson AL, Marsh DJ, Robinson BG: Genetic testing in pheochromocytoma- and paraganglioma-associated syndromes. Ann NY Acad Sci 2006;1073:104–111.
34 Erlic Z, Neumann HP: Diagnosing patients with hereditary paraganglial tumours. Lancet Oncol 2009;10:741.
35 Cascón A, López-Jiménez E, Landa I, Leskelä S, Leandro-García LJ, Maliszewska A, Letón R, de la Vega L, García-Barcina MJ, Sanabria C, Alvarez-Escolá C, Rodríguez-Antona C, Robledo M: Rationalization of genetic testing in patients with apparently sporadic pheochromocytoma/paraganglioma. Horm Metab Res 2009;41:672–675.
36 Bertherat J, Gimenez-Roqueplo AP: New insights in the genetics of adrenocortical tumors, pheochromocytomas and paragangliomas. Horm Metab Res 2005;37:384–390.
37 Burnichon N, Brière JJ, Libé R, Vescovo L, Rivière J, Tissier F, Jouanno E, Jeunemaitre X, Bénit P, Tzagoloff A, Rustin P, Bertherat J, Favier J, Gimenez-Roqueplo AP: SDHA is a tumor suppressor gene causing paraganglioma. Hum Mol Genet 2010;19:3011–3020.
38 Qin Y, Yao L, King EE, Buddavarapu K, Lenci RE, Chocron ES, Lechleiter JD, Sass M, Aronin N, Schiavi F, Boaretto F, Opocher G, Toledo RA, Toledo SP, Stiles C, Aguiar RC, Dahia PL: Germline mutations in TMEM127 confer susceptibility to pheochromocytoma. Nat Genet 2010;42:229–233.
39 Yao L, Schiavi F, Cascon A, Qin Y, Inglada-Pérez L, King EE, Toledo RA, Ercolino T, Rapizzi E, Ricketts CJ, Mori L, Giacchè M, Mendola A, Taschin E, Boaretto F, Loli P, Iacobone M, Rossi GP, Biondi B, Lima-Junior JV, Kater CE, Bex M, Vikkula M, Grossman AB, Gruber SB, Barontini M, Persu A, Castellano M, Toledo SP, Maher ER, Mannelli M, Opocher G, Robledo M, Dahia PL: Spectrum and prevalence of FP/TMEM127 gene mutations in pheochromocytomas and paragangliomas. JAMA 2010;304:2611–2619.

Constantine A. Stratakis
Section on Endocrinology and Genetics
Program on Developmental Endocrinology and Genetics
Eunice Kennedy Shriver National Institute of Child Health and Human Development (NICHD)
31 Center Drive
Bethesda, MD 20892-2425 (USA)

Alford RL, Sutton VR (eds): Medical Genetics in the Clinical Practice of ORL.
Adv Otorhinolaryngol. Basel, Karger, 2011, vol 70, pp 107–113

Genetic Causes of Nonsyndromic Cleft Lip with or without Cleft Palate

Qiuping Yuan[a] · Susan H. Blanton[b] · Jacqueline T. Hecht[a]

[a]Department of Pediatrics, University of Texas Medical School at Houston, Houston, Tex., and [b]University of Miami Miller School of Medicine, Miami, Fla., USA

Abstract

Nonsyndromic cleft lip with or without an associated cleft palate (NSCLP) is one of the most common birth defects affecting 135,000 babies worldwide each year. It causes severe facial dysmorphism and treatment requires a multifaceted team approach. While treatment modalities have improved, the costs to families and the health care resources are still enormous. The causes of NSCLP are multifactorial with both genetic and environmental factors. Progress is being made towards defining the genetic variation underpinning NSCLP by utilizing gene discovery techniques including genome wide linkage, association mapping and a candidate gene approaches. To date, approximately 20% of the genetic contributions to NSCLP have been assigned to a small number of genes. This chapter provides a review of recent progress in defining the genetic causes of NSCLP.

Orofacial clefting is a common birth defect that is most often an isolated anomaly (in 70% of cases); however, in 30% of cases it is associated with other birth defects (syndromic) [1]. The etiology of syndromic clefting can be chromosomal, Mendelian or sporadic [1]. Nonsyndromic cleft lip with or without an associated cleft palate (NSCLP) occurs in 1/700–1,000 newborns with the birth prevalence varying based on geographic origin; it is higher in Asians and lowest in African-Americans (1/500 vs. 1/2,500 births, respectively) [1]. These differences appear to persist even after migration, suggesting that they are mediated by genetic, rather than environmental factors [2]. Males are affected twice as frequently as females; unilateral clefts, with primarily left sided involvement, are more common than bilateral clefts [2]. Problems with feeding, swallowing, speaking and recurrent ear infections are common complications. Multiple surgical repairs, and speech and dental interventions impose substantial economic burdens on the families and society [2].

Twin concordance and family studies provide strong evidence for a genetic basis to NSCLP [1, 2]. The multifactorial model invoking both genetic and environmental factors is favored for NSCLP [1]. Accumulating evidence suggests that environmental factors such as maternal tobacco smoking and maternal folate deficiency are risk factors for NSCLP [1, 2]. Identification of genetic variation contributing to NSCLP has led to an increase in our understanding of the disease process. The results of linkage and genome-wide association studies and candidate gene testing are summarized in table 1 and discussed in the following sections.

Table 1. NSCLP chromosomal regions and genes

Region[1]	Gene	
	CLP phenotype[2]	Association[3]
1p12-13[4]		GSTM1*
1p36	MTHFR (M)	MTHFR*, †, PAX7
1q31.3-q32.2	IRF6 (H&M)	IRF6*, †
2p13		TGFA*, †
2q32-q36	DLX2 (H), SATB2 (H&M), SUMO1 (H&M)	SUMO1
3p21.2	TGFBR2 (H&M), WNT5A (M)	WNT5A†
3q27-q28	TP63 (H&M)	
6p24-p23	EDN1 (M), TFAP2A (H&M)	EDN1
7p15	EGFR (M)	
8p11-p23.3	FGFR1 (H&M), NAT1 (M)	FGFR1, NAT1, NAT2*
9q21-q22	FOXE1 (H&M), PTCH1 (H), TGFBR1 (H)	FOXE1, PTCH1
10q23-q26	FGF8 (H), FGFR2 (H&M)	CYP2E1*
11p12-q14		GSTP1*
14q12	PAX9 (H&M)	PAX9
14q21-q24	BMP4 (H&M), TGFB3 (M)	BMP4*, TGFB3*
15q15	GABRB3 (M)	FGF7, GABRB3
16q12.1-q24	CDH1 (H), FOXC2 (H)	CRISPLD2
17q21	WNT9b (M)	
19p13-q12		BCL3†
19q13.3	CLPTM1 (H&M)	CLPTM1, PVRL2
22q12.2-q12.3		MYH9*
Xcen-q21	EFNB1 (H), TBX22 (H&M)	

[1]Chromosomal region or part of the region reported significant linkage by genome scan studies.
[2]Genes that, when mutated, cause a cleft phenotype in humans (H) or mice (M).
[3]Genes that show a significant association with NSCLP, or gene-environment (*) or gene-gene (†) interaction (or joint effect) in some populations.
[4]Chromosomal regions identified by whole genome scan, that genes have not been found to be associated with NSCLP: 1p31-p21, 1p32.3, 2p16.3, 2q22.3, 2q37, 3p25, 3q24-q26.33, 4q21-q26, 4q28.1, 4q32-q33, 5q11, 6p12.3, 6q14, 6q23-q25, 7p21.3, 7q21, 7q34, 8q11.2-q12, 8q21.3-q24.21, 9p23, 11p11.12, 12p11-q24, 13q33.1-q34, 14q32.32, 15q26, 17q13.1, 18q21.1, 20p12, 20q13.

Genetic Mapping of NSCLP Susceptibility Loci

Linkage analysis in NSCLP has identified regions on all chromosomes, except chromosome 21; however, the results are not consistent between studies (summarized in [3, 4]). Meta-analysis of genome-wide studies from seven populations identified six common chromosomal regions; expansion to thirteen populations found eleven potential disease loci, only two of which, 6q23-q25 and 14q21-q24 overlapped (table 1) [4]. More recently, two genome-wide association studies have found strong evidence for an association to rs987525 in the 8q24 chromosomal region

($p = 3.34 \times 10^{-24}$ and $p = 9.8 \times 10^{-8}$) [5, 6]. This association has been replicated by our group using the same set of single nucleotide polymorphisms (SNPs) ($p = 3.0 \times 10^{-6}$ for rs987525) [7]. However, this region is a gene desert and this association is most likely in linkage disequilibrium (LD) with another causative gene or is a regulatory variant for a gene yet to be identified.

Candidate Gene Screening

Candidate genes for NSCLP are categorized into three broad categories: genes involved in normal craniofacial development including genes causing syndromic CLP, xenobiotic metabolism, and folate metabolism genes.

Developmental Genes

Interferon Regulatory Factor 6 (IRF6). The most significant milestone has been the discovery that variation in *IRF6* gene plays a significant role in NSCLP. Mutations in *IRF6* cause Van der Woude syndrome which is characterized by CLP or cleft palate and/or small pits on the lower lip (OMIM No. 607199). Genome scans of NSCLP have also identified the 1q32-q41 chromosomal region which contains *IRF6* [3]. Numerous studies have validated the *IRF6* association and variation in *IRF6* is estimated to account for approximately 12% of the genetic contribution to NSCLP [8].

A common SNP, rs642961 (G>A), located in the promoter region of *IRF6*, is within an AP2α transcription factor binding site [9]. Substitution of the 'G' allele by 'A' completely eliminates DNA binding. For those with cleft lip only, there was a relative risk of 1.68 for heterozygotes and 2.4 for 'AA' homozygote ($p = 1 \times 10^{-11}$) [9]. Gene interactions between *IRF6* and methylenetetrahydrofolate reductase (MTHFR) and gene-smoking interaction have been reported, suggesting that there is a synergistic effect when two or more risk factors are present [10]. These findings are consistent with the multifactorial model and begin to define a novel NSCLP developmental pathway involving *IRF6*.

Irf6 is a transcription factor that functions as a key determinant for oral epithelial cell differentiation during palatal fusion [11]. Transgenic mice with either Irf6 knockout or the most common Irf6 mutation, R84C (arginine to cystine amino acid change at position 84), show abnormal skin, limbs and craniofacial development including cleft palate [11, 12]. Expression of Irf6 colocalizes with transforming growth factor Tgfbr2 in the medial edge epithelia (MEE) during palatal formation and is downregulated in the Tgfbr2 null mutant mice, suggesting that Tgfbr2 signaling mediates Irf6 expression [13].

Cysteine-Rich Secretory Protein LCCL Domain Containing 2 (CRISPLD2). Genome scan studies identified the 16q22–24 chromosomal region as potentially containing a clefting gene (table 1) [14]. CRISPLD2 (also known as Lgl1) is a secreted glycoprotein and functions as a major modulator in early branching morphogenesis of the developing lung and kidney. Significant association was found for the SNP rs1546124 in *CRISPLD2* and for haplotypes composed of SNPs rs1546124 with either rs4783099 or rs16974880 in the non-Hispanic white families and rs8061351 with rs2326398 in the Hispanic families [15]. Expression of CRISPLD2 was detected in the mandible, nasal and palatal regions of E12.5–E17.5 mouse embryos which spans the critical stages of lip/palatal formation [15]. These results show that *CRISPLD2* is another important NSCLP gene and is involved in lip/palatal development.

MSX1. MSX1 is a transcriptional repressor [1, 3]. Msx1-deficient mice have multiple craniofacial defects including a clefting secondary palate, abnormalities of several facial bones and tooth agenesis [1]. In humans, mutations in *MSX1* cause selective tooth agenesis (STHAG1) syndrome (OMIM No. 106600), which is characterized by absence of the premolars and third molars (wisdom teeth), with some cases displaying oral clefts. A nonsense mutation in *MSX1* co-segregates with tooth agenesis and oral clefts in a three-generation Dutch family [1]. In a Dutch case-control study, homozygosity for allele 4 of a microsatellite marker in the *MSX1* gene conferred a 2.7-fold higher risk of having oral clefts when the mother smoked during pregnancy. The risk increased about 5-fold when both parents smoked [16]. Maternal homozygosity for this allele and smoking also increased the risk [16]. Jezewski et al. (Reviewed in [3]) sequenced *MSX1* gene in NSCLP cases and controls and rare variants were found in approximately 2% of NSCLP cases. MSX1 may play a causal role in a small subset of NSCLP patients.

Fibroblast Growth Factor (FGF) Signal Pathway. FGFs and their receptors (FGFRs) comprise a large, complex signaling pathway important in embryogenesis and tissue homeostasis [17]. Fgf8, Fgf10, Fgfr2b and Fgfr1 knockout mice have cleft lip/palate [17]. In humans, loss-of-function mutations in *FGF8* and *FGF10* cause NSCLP, and loss-of-functions in the FGF receptors, FGFR1, FGFR2 and FGFR3, cause syndromic forms of CLP. Associations have been reported between *FGF3*, *FGF7*, *FGF10*, *FGF18* and *FGFR1* and NSCLP. Sequencing of the coding regions of *FGF8*, *FGF10*, *FGFR1*, *FGFR2* and *FGFR3* in NSCLP cases identified eight missense variations, six of which, were not present in the controls. These results suggest that rare coding sequence variant may contribute to a small number of NSCLP cases.

WNT Signal Pathways. Mutations in *WNT3* in humans cause tetra-amelia syndrome (OMIM No. 273395), a severe recessive birth malformation characterized by absence of all four limbs and other anomalies including CLP. Wnt9b knockout mice have lethal malformations and CLP (OMIM No. 602864). Significant associations between *WNT3A*, *WNT5A*, *WNT8A* and *WNT11* and NSCLP, were found in non-Hispanic white and Hispanic families but not with *WNT3* and *WNT9B* [18]. These results suggest that WNT3 and WNT9B are not important in human NSCLP in the populations tested; however, other WNT genes may play a role in NSCLP.

TGFs Signal Pathways. Transforming growth factors (TGFs), including TGFA, TGFBs and bone morphogenetic proteins (BMPs), belong to a large family of hormonal proteins that regulate cell proliferation, differentiation, migration and apoptosis [19]. A cleft lip and/or palate phenotype results when Tgfs and receptors, including Egfr (epidermal growth factor receptor, a putative receptor of Tgfa), Tgfb3 and its receptors Tgfr1, Tgfr2, Bmp4, Bmp11 and their receptors Alk2 and Alk3, are knocked out in mice [20–22]. Expression of mouse Tgfa and Tgfb3 has been detected during palatal fusion [1].

Ardinger et al. (Reviewed in [1]) first reported an association between the TaqI variant in *TGFA* with NSCLP, and later, an association with *TGFB3*. Both *TGFA* and *TGFB3* have been extensively interrogated for linkage, association and gene-environment interactions with inconsistent results.

Other Developmental Genes. The myosin heavy chain 9, non muscle *(MYH9)* gene encodes a myosin IIA heavy chain subunit, which is involved in cytokinesis, cell motility and maintenance of cell shape; it is highly expressed in the palatal shelves before fusion [23]. Significant association was found between common variants in *MYH9* and NSCLP [24, 25]. One study found interaction between maternal passive smoking and homozygosity for the rs16996652 T allele, which conferred a two-fold higher risk for NSCLP [24].

Small ubiquitin-related modifier (*SUMO1*) is strongly expressed in the upper lip, primary palate and MEE of the secondary palate [26]. This gene was identified as a potential candidate when a t(2;8)(q33.1;q24.3) chromosomal translocation was identified in a 5-year-old girl with unilateral CLP [26]. The breakpoint of this translocation on 2q maps to intron 2 of the *SUMO1* gene and interrupts the gene [26]. Further, mice with Sumo1 haploinsufficiency (Sumo1$^{+/-}$) have cleft palate [26]. Two recent studies also found an association between gene variations in *SUMO1* and NSCLP

[28, 29]. *SUMO1* has subsequently been found to play a role in posttranslational modification of several proteins associated with NSCLP: the tumor protein TP63, MSX1, PAX9 (paired box 9), SATB2 (SATB homeobox 2), TBX22 (T-box 22) and Eya1 (eyes absent homolog 1) [26, 29]. These findings place SUMO1 in a novel molecular pathway relevant to the pathogenesis of NSCLP.

Rare mutations have been found in a few other genes, *FOXE1* (forkhead box E1), *GLI2* (GLI family zinc finger 2), *JAG2* (Jagged2), *LHX8* (LIM homeobox 8), *MSX2*, (*SATB2*), *SKI* (ski sarcoma viral oncogene homolog), *SPRY2* (sprouty homolog 2) and *TBX10* (T-box 10), and may contribute to a small number of NSCLP cases [30].

Detoxification Genes

Several studies have evaluated the maternal and fetal null genotypes with respect to prenatal smoke exposure and NSCLP and three studies reported joint effects between maternal smoking and *GSTM1* and *GSTT1* null genotypes [21]. For example, maternal smoking in combination with a fetus lacking GSTM1 activity conferred a 7-fold increased risk of NSCLP when the mother smoked 20 cigarettes per day [31]. Another study found that prenatal exposure to 1–4, 5–14 or ≥15 cigarette/day fetus' with the *GSTT1*-null genotype increased the risk of NSCLP 2-, 6- and 17-fold, respectively [32].

Other genes participating in the detoxification cascade have also been assessed [21]. Genetic variants in several genes, *CYP1A1* and *CYP2E1* (cytochrome P450 proteins), *EPHX1* (epoxide hydrolase 1), *GSTP1* (glutathione S-transferase P1) and *HIF1* (hypoxia-induced factor), were found to interact with maternal smoking producing a synergistic risk effect for NSCLP [21]. However, conflicting results have been reported in other studies [21].

Folate Metabolic Genes

Periconceptional folic acid supplementation has been shown to reduce the recurrence of NSCLP in families and in mice [33]. This has led to interrogation of genes in the folate metabolism pathway in NSCLP families. The common mutation C677T in *MTHFR* converts alanine to valine and results in reduced enzyme activity and elevated plasma homocysteine level and is a risk factor for neural tube defects and coronary heart disease [34]. Numerous studies and meta-analyses have assessed C677T and other variants in *MTHFR* and few have found an association with NSCLP [33, 35].

We have recently interrogated 14 folate metabolism-related genes in multiplex and simplex non-Hispanic white and Hispanic NSCLP families [Blanton et al., 2010, in press]. Evidence for association between NSCLP and variants in *NOS3* and *TYMS* (thymidylate synthetase) was detected in the non-Hispanic white group, whereas associations with *MTR*, *BHMT2*, *MTHFS* (5,10-methenyltetrahydrofolate synthetase) and *SLC19A1* were detected in the Hispanic group [Blanton et al., 2010, in press]. Of particular interest were the interactions between SNPs in *CBS* and SNPs in *BHMT2*, *FOLR1*, *FOLR2* (folate receptor 1 and 2), *MTHFD1* (methylenetetrahydrofolate dehydrogenase), *MTHFR*, *MTRR*, *NOS3*, *SLC19A1* and *TYMS* suggesting that perturbations of the genes in the folate pathway, and particularly, the methionine arm, contribute to NSCLP. Similarly, two previously published studies from the same group investigated 9 and 29 folate genes using the same Norwegian NSCLP triads [36, 37]. Associations were found for rs234706 in *CBS* in the first study, while in the latter study, associations to three SNPs in *DMGDH* (dimethylglycine dehydrogenase), (rs479405, rs1805074 and rs532964) and two SNPs in *CBS* (rs234705 and rs4920037) were reported. Other studies have also found an association between NSCLP and genes in the methionine metabolic arm, including *MTHFD1*, *MTR* and *CBS* [38–40]. Shaw et al. [38] observed joint effects between the infant *NOS3* variants and maternal smoking with a 4-fold higher risk for the infants if the mother did not take vitamins during early pregnancy. Despite different study designs in different populations, *CBS* has consistently been associated with NSCLP [36, 37, 40, 41]. Overall, these results provide evidence that perturbation of genes in the methionine arm of the folate pathway may play a causal role in NSCLP.

Conclusions

NSCLP is a complex disorder that is caused by the consequence of actions and interactions of many genetic and environmental factors and these will likely differ between populations. Use of a variety of genetic approaches has identified approximately 20% of the genetic variation contributing to NSCLP but much work remains to be done before high-risk haplotypes are identified and risk models are developed that can be used in risk assessment and population screening.

References

1 Murray JC: Gene/environment causes of cleft lip and/or palate. Clin Genet 2002; 61:248–256.
2 Bender PL: Genetics of cleft lip and palate. J Pediatr Nurs 2000;15:242–249.
3 Lidral AC, Moreno LM: Progress toward discerning the genetics of cleft lip. Curr Opin Pediatr 2005;17:731–739.
4 Marazita ML, Murray JC, Lidral AC, et al: Meta-analysis of 13 genome scans reveals multiple cleft lip/palate genes with novel loci on 9q21 and 2q32–35. Am J Hum Genet 2004;75:161–173.
5 Grant SF, Wang K, Zhang H, Glaberson W, Annaiah K, Kim CE, Bradfield JP, Glessner JT, Thomas KA, Garris M, Frackelton EC, Otieno FG, Chiavacci RM, Nah HD, Kirschner RE, Hakonarson H: A genome-wide association study identifies a locus for nonsyndromic cleft lip with or without cleft palate on 8q24. J Pediatr 2009;155:909–913.
6 Birnbaum S, Ludwig KU, Reutter H, Herms S, Steffens M, Rubini M, Baluardo C, Ferrian M, Almeida de Assis N, Alblas MA, Barth S, Freudenberg J, Lauster C, Schmidt G, Scheer M, Braumann B, Bergé SJ, Reich RH, Schiefke F, Hemprich A, Pötzsch S, Steegers-Theunissen RP, Pötzsch B, Moebus S, Horsthemke B, Kramer FJ, Wienker TF, Mossey PA, Propping P, Cichon S, Hoffmann P, Knapp M, Nöthen MM, Mangold E: Key susceptibility locus for nonsyndromic cleft lip with or without cleft palate on chromosome 8q24. Nat Genet 2009;41:473–477.
7 Blanton SH, Burt A, Stal S, Mulliken JB, Garcia E, Hecht JT: Family-based study shows heterogeneity of a susceptibility locus on chromosome 8q24 for nonsyndromic cleft lip and palate. Birth Defects Res A Clin Mol Teratol 2010;88:256–259.
8 Zucchero TM, Cooper ME, Maher BS, et al: Interferon regulatory factor 6 (IRF6) gene variants and the risk of isolated cleft lip or palate. N Engl J Med 2004; 351:769–780.
9 Rahimov F, Marazita ML, Visel A, et al: Disruption of an AP-2alpha binding site in an IRF6 enhancer is associated with cleft lip. Nat Genet 2008;40:1341–1347.
10 Ali A, Singh SK, Raman R: MTHFR 677TT alone and IRF6 820GG together with MTHFR 677CT, but not MTHFR A1298C, are risks for nonsyndromic cleft lip with or without cleft palate in an Indian population. Genet Test Mol Biomarkers 2009;13:355–360.
11 Richardson RJ, Dixon J, Malhotra S, Hardman MJ, Knowles L, Boot-Handford RP, Shore P, Whitmarsh A, Dixon MJ: Irf6 is a key determinant of the keratinocyte proliferation-differentiation switch. Nat Genet 2006; 38:1329–1334.
12 Ingraham CR, Kinoshita A, Kondo S, Yang B, Sajan S, Trout KJ, Malik MI, Dunnwald M, Goudy SL, Lovett M, Murray JC, Schutte BC: Abnormal skin, limb and craniofacial morphogenesis in mice deficient for interferon regulatory factor 6 (Irf6). Nat Genet 2006;38:1335–1340.
13 Xu X, Han J, Ito Y, Bringas P Jr, Urata MM, Chai Y: Cell autonomous requirement for Tgfbr2 in the disappearance of medial edge epithelium during palatal fusion. Dev Biol 2006;297:238–248.
14 Vieira AR, McHenry TG, Daack-Hirsch S, Murray JC, Marazita ML: A genome wide linkage scan for cleft lip and palate and dental anomalies. Am J Med Genet A 2008;146A:1406–1413.
15 Chiquet BT, Lidral AC, Stal S, Mulliken JB, Moreno LM, Arcos-Burgos M, Valencia-Ramirez C, Blanton SH, Hecht JT: CRISPLD2: a novel NSCLP candidate gene. Hum Mol Genet 2007;16:2241–2248.
16 van den Boogaard MJ, de Costa D, Krapels IP, Liu F, van Duijn C, Sinke RJ, Lindhout D, Steegers-Theunissen RP: The MSX1 allele 4 homozygous child exposed to smoking at periconception is most sensitive in developing nonsyndromic orofacial clefts. Hum Genet 2008; 124:525–534.
17 Krejci P, Prochazkova J, Bryja V, Kozubik A, Wilcox WR: Molecular pathology of the fibroblast growth factor family. Hum Mutat 2009;30:1245–1255.
18 Chiquet BT, Blanton SH, Burt A, Ma D, Stal S, Mulliken JB, Hecht JT: Variation in WNT genes is associated with nonsyndromic cleft lip with or without cleft palate. Hum Mol Genet 2008;17:2212–2218.
19 Wu MY, Hill CS: Tgf-beta superfamily signaling in embryonic development and homeostasis. Dev Cell 2009;16:329–343.

20 Nie X, Luukko K, Kettunen P: BMP signalling in craniofacial development. Int J Dev Biol 2006;50:511–521.
21 Shi M, Wehby GL, Murray JC: Review on genetic variants and maternal smoking in the etiology of oral clefts and other birth defects. Birth Defects Res C Embryo Today 2008;84:16–29.
22 Stanier P, Moore GE: Genetics of cleft lip and palate: syndromic genes contribute to the incidence of non-syndromic clefts. Hum Mol Genet 2004;13:R73–R81.
23 Zang JH, Cavet G, Sabry JH, Wagner P, Moores SL, Spudich JA: On the role of myosin-II in cytokinesis: division of *Dictyostelium* cells under adhesive and nonadhesive conditions. Mol Biol Cell 1997;8:2617–2629.
24 Jia ZL, Li Y, Chen CH, Li S, Wang Y, Zheng Q, Shi B: Association among polymorphisms at MYH9, environmental factors, and nonsyndromic orofacial clefts in western China. DNA Cell Biol 2010;29:25–32.
25 Chiquet BT, Hashmi SS, Henry R, Burt A, Mulliken JB, Stal S, Bray M, Blanton SH, Hecht JT: Genomic screening identifies novel linkages and provides further evidence for a role of MYH9 in nonsyndromic cleft lip and palate. Eur J Hum Genet 2009;17:195–204.
26 Alkuraya FS, Saadi I, Lund JJ, Turbe-Doan A, Morton CC, Maas RL: SUMO1 haploinsufficiency leads to cleft lip and palate. Science 2006;313:1751.
27 Song T, Li G, Jing G, Jiao X, Shi J, Zhang B, Wang L, Ye X, Cao F: SUMO1 polymorphisms are associated with non-syndromic cleft lip with or without cleft palate. Biochem Biophys Res Commun 2008;377:1265–1268.
28 Carter TC, Molloy AM, Pangilinan F, Troendle JF, Kirke PN, Conley MR, Orr DJ, Earley M, McKiernan E, Lynn EC, Doyle A, Scott JM, Brody LC, Mills JL: Testing reported associations of genetic risk factors for oral clefts in a large Irish study population. Birth Defects Res A Clin Mol Teratol 2010;88:84–93.
29 Pauws E, Stanier P: FGF signalling and SUMO modification: new players in the aetiology of cleft lip and/or palate. Trends Genet 2007;23:631–640.
30 Vieira AR, Avila JR, Daack-Hirsch S, Dragan E, Felix TM, Rahimov F, Harrington J, Schultz RR, Watanabe Y, Johnson M, Fang J, O'Brien SE, Orioli IM, Castilla EE, Fitzpatrick DR, Jiang R, Marazita ML, Murray JC: Medical sequencing of candidate genes for nonsyndromic cleft lip and palate. PLoS Genet 2005;1:e64.
31 Lammer EJ, Shaw GM, Iovannisci DM, Finnell RH: Maternal smoking, genetic variation of glutathione s-transferases, and risk for orofacial clefts. Epidemiology 2005;16:698–701.
32 Shi M, Christensen K, Weinberg CR, Romitti P, Bathum L, Lozada A, Morris RW, Lovett M, Murray JC: Orofacial cleft risk is increased with maternal smoking and specific detoxification-gene variants. Am J Hum Genet 2007;80:76–90.
33 Wehby GL, Murray JC: Folic acid and orofacial clefts: a review of the evidence. Oral Dis 2010;16:11–19.
34 Beaudin AE, Stover PJ: Folate-mediated one-carbon metabolism and neural tube defects: balancing genome synthesis and gene expression. Birth Defects Res C Embryo Today 2007;81:183–203.
35 Verkleij-Hagoort A, Bliek J, Sayed-Tabatabaei F, Ursem N, Steegers E, Steegers-Theunissen R: Hyperhomocysteinemia and MTHFR polymorphisms in association with orofacial clefts and congenital heart defects: a meta-analysis. Am J Med Genet A 2007;143A:952–960.
36 Boyles AL, Wilcox AJ, Taylor JA, Meyer K, Fredriksen A, Ueland PM, Drevon CA, Vollset SE, Lie RT: Folate and one-carbon metabolism gene polymorphisms and their associations with oral facial clefts. Am J Med Genet A 2008; 146A:440–449.
37 Boyles AL, Wilcox AJ, Taylor JA, Shi M, Weinberg CR, Meyer K, Fredriksen A, Ueland PM, Johansen AM, Drevon CA, Jugessur A, Trung TN, Gjessing HK, Vollset SE, Murray JC, Christensen K, Lie RT: Oral facial clefts and gene polymorphisms in metabolism of folate/one-carbon and vitamin A: a pathway-wide association study. Genet Epidemiol 2009;33:247–255.
38 Mills JL, Molloy AM, Parle-McDermott A, Troendle JF, Brody LC, Conley MR, Cox C, Pangilinan F, Orr DJ, Earley M, McKiernan E, Lynn EC, Doyle A, Scott JM, Kirke PN: Folate-related gene polymorphisms as risk factors for cleft lip and cleft palate. Birth Defects Res A Clin Mol Teratol 2008;82:636–643.
39 Mostowska A, Hozyasz KK, Jagodzinski PP: Maternal MTR genotype contributes to the risk of non-syndromic cleft lip and palate in the Polish population. Clin Genet 2006;69:512–517.
40 Rubini M, Brusati R, Garattini G, Magnani C, Liviero F, Bianchi F, Tarantino E, Massei A, Pollastri S, Carturan S, Amadori A, Bertagnin E, Cavallaro A, Fabiano A, Franchella A, Calzolari E: Cystathionine beta-synthase c.844ins68 gene variant and non-syndromic cleft lip and palate. Am J Med Genet A 2005;136A:368–372.
41 Shaw GM, Iovannisci DM, Yang W, Finnell RH, Carmichael SL, Cheng S, Lammer EJ: Endothelial nitric oxide synthase (NOS3) genetic variants, maternal smoking, vitamin use, and risk of human orofacial clefts. Am J Epidemiol 2005;162:1207–1214.

Jacqueline T. Hecht, PhD
University of Texas Medical School at Houston, Department of Pediatrics
6431 Fannin Street, Ste 3.136
Houston, TX 77030 (USA)
Tel. +1 713 500 5764, Fax +1 713 500 5689, E-Mail Jacqueline.T.Hecht@uth.tmc.edu

Alford RL, Sutton VR (eds): Medical Genetics in the Clinical Practice of ORL.
Adv Otorhinolaryngol. Basel, Karger, 2011, vol 70, pp 114–121

Chronic Rhinosinusitis

Xinjing Wang[a] · Garry R. Cutting[b]

National Eye Institute, National Institutes of Health, Bethesda, Md., and Johns Hopkins Medical Institutes, Baltimore, Md., USA

Abstract

Chronic rhinosinusitis (CRS) is a persistent inflammatory condition involving the nasal and paranasal mucosa. It is the most prevalent chronic condition in the United States. Sinonasal inflammation is also a common clinical presentation in a variety of systemic conditions. The etiology of CRS is complicated as a variety of extrinsic and intrinsic factors are frequently involved. Extrinsic factors include microbial infections that trigger abnormal immune responses. Intrinsic factors may predispose an individual to infection or exaggerated inflammatory responses. Several systemic conditions such as cystic fibrosis (CF), primary ciliary dyskinesia (PCD), asthma, immunohyperresponsiveness, and immunodeficiencies illustrate the role of genetic abnormalities in the development of CRS. Both common and rare genetic variants have been found in an association with CRS. A role for genetic factors is also supported by the demonstration of CRS clustering in families. Although the majority of CRS cases are considered to be idiopathic, the pathological evidence suggests that the chronic condition could be an overlapped presentation of multiple underlying mechanisms. Systemic conditions may have an impact on the incidence, severity, prognosis, or treatment of patients with CRS. Evaluation for underlying conditions may help the otolaryngologist manage the symptoms of CRS and optimize therapy.

Almost all humans have experienced nasal infections during their lifetime. Acute rhinosinusitis can develop as an inflammatory complication of an upper respiratory tract infection caused by rhinoviruses or other acute conditions. Viral infection by itself does not appear to cause progression to chronic nasal conditions as complete recovery generally occurs in 99% of individuals. However, individuals may develop secondary sinonasal infections from prior viral infection. Most prolonged cases of rhinosinusitis can be successfully treated with appropriate antimicrobial medication.

Chronic rhinosinusitis (CRS) refers to a persistent inflammation involving the nasal and paranasal mucosa. It can evolve from acute infection, but many individuals with chronic nasal and paranasal inflammation do not have a preceding acute phase [1]. Some patients have recurrent acute episodes despite successful treatment of prior episodes [2]. Therefore, CRS does not appear to be a simple progression of acute infection. This chapter will review the extrinsic and intrinsic contributing factors in the pathological process of CRS and the systemic conditions that may affect the incidence, severity and prognosis of CRS with emphasis on the genetic contributions.

Chronic Rhinosinusitis and Clinical Evaluations

Prevalence, Clinical Presentations, and Extrinsic Factors

CRS is the most prevalent chronic condition in the United States. Two National Health Interview

Table 1. Symptoms for diagnosis of chronic rhinosinusitis

Major symptoms	Minor symptoms
Nasal discharge (anterior or posterior)	headache
Nasal obstruction	ear pain-pressure-fullness
Facial congestion	halitosis
Facial pain-pressure-fullness	dental pain
Hyposmia-anosmia	cough
	fever
	fatigue

CRS diagnosis requires 12 weeks affected time with ≥ two major symptoms or 12 weeks affected time with one major symptom plus ≥ two minor symptoms. Adapted from Meltzer et al. [5].

Surveys found the prevalence at 141.3 per 1,000 persons and 125.5 per 1,000 persons in the population [3, 4]. Millions of dollars are spent on treatment every year [3]. CRS is commonly diagnosed using patient history and physical examination. According to current consensus diagnostic criteria in general practice, CRS clinical presentation includes major and minor symptoms [5], and patients presenting with either two major symptoms or one major with two minor symptoms for 12 or more weeks are considered to have CRS [5–7] (table 1). Patients usually present with several or all symptoms with variable severities [2]. CRS may not have a single etiology since many risk factors have been identified [5]. The most common causative extrinsic pathogen is microorganism infection. Community-acquired bacteria, anaerobes, odontogenic oral microflora, and fungi are all present in the nasal secretions of CRS patients [5, 8]. However, these microorganisms can also be isolated from individuals without sinus symptoms [9]. Exposure to extrinsic microorganisms may not necessarily and sufficiently lead to chronic infection such as to form biofilms or lead to osteitis. Cigarette smoke exposure, pollutants and allergens are also possible extrinsic factors. These factors may only be associated with abnormal responses in the adaptive immune system or impairments in respiratory epithelial function, leading to CRS. These impairments and abnormal responses to extrinsic factors may be due to either gene-environment interaction or to intrinsic factors [10].

Pathology and Intrinsic Factors

The structural and functional integrity of nose and paranasal sinuses depends on intact innate and adaptive immunities, normal mucus blanket, normal mucociliary clearance, patent sinonasal drainage pathways, supportive blood vessels, and regulatory nervous system. Pathological evidence has been found in each aspect of these normal physiological processes in CRS patients [5]. Eosinophilia, neutrophilia, and overexpressed cytokines or chemokines within the immune system signaling pathways in individuals with CRS suggest that abnormal immune responses are intrinsic contributing factors [5, 11]. Extensive genomic studies of genes in the immune components such as the complement factors, leukotriene synthases and interleukin receptors have correlated many gene variants with susceptibility to acquired abnormal immune responses [12–15]. Gene variants may contribute to CRS as monogenic diseases, complex disorders, or as gene-environment interactions. Monogenic diseases such as CF and PCD have single gene mutations responsible for abnormal mucociliary clearance and immune response [16, 17]. Allergy, asthma and chronic sinusitis are associated as a complex disorder. Multiple underlying mechanisms might simultaneously contribute to the development of allergic rhinitis, asthma and CRS [18]. Smoking may complicate the development and treatment of CRS [19, 20]. Bartoloni et al. [21] reported a patient who may have overlapped presentation of sinus abnormality from multiple underlying mechanisms. The patient had situs inversus totalis and CF. He was homozygous for *CFTR* mutation ΔF508 because of uniparental disomy of chromosome 7. The patient was also identified with ciliary defects and diagnosed with Kartagener syndrome. They found a homozygous nonsense mutation in the *DNAH11* gene on the short arm of chromosome 7. The *DNAH11* and *CFTR* mutations segregated in this patient, leading to more severe respiratory symptoms. In this chapter, these genetic contributions will be discussed in the context of related systemic conditions.

Patients with Chronic Rhinosinusitis and Systemic Conditions

Chronic Rhinosinusitis in Patients with Abnormal Immune System

Allergic Rhinitis, Sinusitis, and Asthma

Allergic rhinitis and asthma are common clinical disorders. The association between allergy, asthma and chronic sinusitis has been recognized for more than a century. Allergic rhinitis, sinusitis, and asthma are likely part of one disease process [18]. The etiology of asthma is at least as complicated as CRS [22, 23]. Genetic studies of asthma revealed numerous loci and complicated inheritance [23–25]. Multiple underlying mechanisms might simultaneously lead to allergic rhinitis, asthma and CRS [18].

Samter's Syndrome

Samter's syndrome is an aspirin-exacerbated respiratory disease. It describes a triad (Samter triad) of nasal polyps with CRS, aspirin-intolerance and asthma [26]. In the incomplete triads, nasal polyposis could be the first clinical symptom [27]. Ingestion of aspirin or several other nonsteroidal anti-inflammation drugs (NSAIDs) exacerbates asthma and rhinosinusitis. The defect is a blockade of the arachidonic acid metabolism pathway, leading to bronchoconstriction and inflammation. The etiology is not clear. Several genomic polymorphisms have been analyzed for genetic association. A polymorphism in the promoter region of leukotriene C4 synthease (LTC4S-444A>C) was identified as a marker for the severe glucocorticoid-dependent phenotype of aspirin-induced asthma [28]. About 20% of all patients with CRS and polyps have aspirin sensitivity [29]. Aspirin desensitization, inhalers, and systemic steroids are used to control the condition. Otological presentations including hearing loss are frequently observed and could be prevented by steroids [27].

Immunodeficiencies

Sinusitis presents in patients with a variety of immunodeficiencies. Opportunistic infections are frequently observed in HIV positive individuals and post-transplantation patients. Local secretory or systemic humoral immunodeficiencies are the most important in this pathogenesis. Humoral immunodeficiency is not uncommon in patients with refractory CRS. Common variable immunodeficiency (CVID) is a group of primary immunodeficiencies with variable low levels of immunoglobins and autoimmunity. Approximately 70 to 80% of these patients have had recurrent sinopulmonary infections [30]. Genetic predispositions, repeated antigen exposures, and immune dysregulation may be the causative factors [31]. The prevalence of CVID is estimated between one in 25,000 and one in 66,000 [32]. The rare X-linked lymphoproliferative diseases are genetically different from CVID [33].

Chronic Rhinosinusitis in Congenital Abnormalities of Epithelial Cells

Chronic Rhinosinusitis in Patients with Cystic Fibrosis

CF is the most common life-threatening autosomal-recessive disorder in the white population, with disease incidence of one in 2,000–4,000 live births and a disease prevalence of approximately 30,000 affected individuals in the US population

[34, 35]. The CF carrier frequency is approximately one in 28 in the North American white population [34]. CF clinical presentation includes sino-pulmonary phenotypes [36]. Chronic inflammation of sinuses and nasal mucosa starts in very early stage of the disease and is extremely common in all CF patients [17]. The cystic fibrosis transmembrane regulator gene *(CFTR)* is responsible for CF. Mutation of CFTR protein, a chloride channel, disrupts epithelial chloride transport, and leads to abnormal ciliary clearance and immunopathological changes. More than 1600 mutations in the *CFTR* gene have been found in CF patients (CFTR mutation database: www.genet.sickkids.on.ca/cftr/). Type of CF mutation, genetic modifiers, and environmental factors contribute to the variation in disease clinical presentations [34, 37, 38]. More *CFTR* gene variations were also found, but did not segregate with typical CF presentations. These gene changes are not considered to be CF mutations. Some CF mutations were found with atypical clinical presentation of CF because there was an incomplete penetrance of those CF mutations [34]. Atypical CF patients often present with CRS for some time without clear systemic conditions of CF, and the CF diagnosis was based on laboratory evidence such as positive genetic testing, positive nasal potential differences and family history [35]. Atypical CF patients were found among regular CRS patients in several studies [39–41].

Chronic Rhinosinusitis in CF Mutation Carriers

The spectrum of CF clinical presentation is broad. Recent studies found that CFTRopathy is not confined to individuals with two mutant alleles [42]. A higher frequency of CF alleles was found in allergic bronchopulmonary aspergillosis patients [43]. In a case-control study with 147 patients with CRS and 123 sinus disease-free controls, nearly 7% of CRS patients carried a CF mutation [39]. Studies on obligate CF carriers by a survey questionnaire and mutation distribution analysis in Maryland and the surrounding area observed that the chronic sinus condition was more frequent than in the general population (36 vs. 14%) [44]. Several other studies also suggested that CF carriers had higher risk of nasal polyps, chronic sinusitis, and disseminated brochiectasis [45–47].

Based on the estimated carrier frequency in North Americans, there are about 9 million CF carriers in the United States. Most likely, CF carriers are suspected and identified because of family history. More and more CF carriers without family history will be identified because of the newborn screening programs and prenatal genetic testing for CF. The question is how the sinus problem was taken care of in a family member of a CF patient after the exclusion of a CF diagnosis. Should the CF carriers be treated differently for their sinus problem? Is there an advantage in adapting some of the CF treatment strategies for CF carriers? It is too early to suggest CF mutation screening in regular CRS patients, but a clinical study of the potential benefit of screening and a unique treatment will be worthwhile.

Chronic Rhinosinusitis in Patients with Primary Ciliary Dyskinesia

PCD refers to a genetically heterogeneous disorder characterized by sino-pulmonary manifestations, usually segregating as autosomal recessive inheritance [48]. It was reported that 1 in 20,000 to 1 in 60,000 live births were diagnosed with PCD [49]. Kartagener syndrome defines the PCD patients who also have laterality defects. Diagnosis of PCD is challenging because it requires a compatible clinical phenotype with ciliary ultrastructural analysis, immunofluorescent analysis, or functional analysis [49, 50]. Mutations in eight genes have been reported in PCD patients [16, 48]. More loci have been identified [51]. Mutations in the *DNAH5* and *DNAI1* genes were found in about 25% to 38% of PCD patients [48, 52]. The frequency of situs inversus was about 1 in 8,000 in the population [53], therefore it would be reasonable to expect a higher frequency of PCD since about 50% of patients would not have laterality defects just by chance. For example, Ng et al. [54] recently reported *DNAH5* gene mutations in a study by exome sequencing on Miller syndrome (postaxial acrofacial dysostosis syndrome) patients. They identified the gene *(DHODH)* for Miller Syndrome in six families, but in one family, they found coexisting *DNAH5* mutations, underlying PCD. Interestingly, affected siblings in this family had been treated in a CF clinic for sinopulmonary conditions. Coste et al. [40] analyzed a cohort of 42 adult patients with severe chronic sinusitis for CFTR mutations and PCD. They found three atypical CF patients (7%) and a higher frequency of CF mutation carriers (19%). They also found equivalently high PCD patients (17%) in this cohort. None of the CF patients or carriers in this cohort is concurrently with a PCD diagnosis. The question is when CRS patients should be evaluated for CF mutation or ciliary function for a potential diagnosis of PCD. No reports were found in the literature describing sinus problem in PCD mutation carriers.

Chronic Rhinosinusitis in Patients with Systemic Vasculitides

The systemic vasculitides are heterogeneous disorders with a primary process of inflammation and damage of blood vessel walls. Wegener's granulomatosis and Churg-Strauss syndrome belong to a group of systemic vasculitides characterized by affecting small-to-medium-sized vessels, and are associated with anti-neutrophil cytoplasmic antibodies [55]. The pulmonary system may be involved in all systemic vasculitides, but anti-neutrophil cytoplasmic antibody-associated systemic vasculitides have much higher frequencies of respiratory involvement such as asthma, sinus inflammation, and subglottic stenosis [56, 57]. The etiology of systemic vasculitides is still unknown, but a complex interaction including genetic contribution is probably involved based on familial clusters and immunogenetic studies [55].

Chronic Rhinosinusitis in Patients with Sinonasal Anatomic Variants

Nasal obstruction is one of the major symptoms in patients with CRS. It was a general belief in textbooks that abnormal airflow leads to crusting and infection [58]. However, complete abolition of nasal airflow through procedures such as laryngectomy did not lead to rhinosinusitis [59]. Nasal septal deviation, concha bullosa, and inferior turbinate enlargement also did not correlate with CRS [59–61]. CRS may be associated with nasal neoplasm. Sino-orbital osteoma was reported as the most common sinus tumor, and CT scan could find osteoma in as much as 3% in the population [62]. Osteomas are benign and slow-growing tumors [63]. Most osteomas are clinically silent. Symptomatic sino-orbital osteoma patients should be evaluated for Gardner's syndrome, a genetic disorder predisposing to colorectal cancer [64]. Concerning neoplasms, refractory CRS should be actively evaluated because prompt diagnosis and treatment may be lifesaving [65].

Hearing Loss and Chronic Rhinosinusitis

Hearing loss was described in detail in the chapter by Lin and Oghalai [this vol.]. It affects 6–8% of the population in developed countries [66]. Rhinogenic deafness correlates with pharyngitis, rhinitis, laryngitis, chronic catarrhalis otitis and CRS. Genetic defects account for approximately 60% of childhood deafness and are correlated with scores of genes [67]. Mutations in the *GJB2* (*CX26*) gene (connexin 26) are the most common hearing loss-causing alleles [68]. BuSaba et al. [69] analyzed 46 consecutive CRS or recurrent acute rhinosinusitis patients for mutations in the *CX26* and connexin 30 (*CX30*) genes. They found no mutations in the *CX30* gene and equivalent frequencies of *CX26* mutation carriers in this cohort. A possible role for mutations in genes other than *CX26* and *CX30* needs to be further examined. Preventing hearing loss as a complication of nasal inflammation is very important for patient care [70].

Current Directions in Genetic Research

The etiology of CRS is not clear. CRS may be associated with multiple independent factors. Since multiple mechanisms may simultaneously lead to CRS, molecular dissection of primary defects may piece together the puzzle. Most important, large scale familial segregation analysis by twin and family studies may provide evidence of genetic contributions. Prospective clinical recruitment of patients with carefully defined diagnoses offers a better approach [5]. Clinical presentations and pathological evidence may not be necessarily different in CRS patients with one primary defect versus another at a single time point. Clinical follow-up and collaborative studies with large recruitment size may provide appropriate categorization of CRS patients for genomewide association scans, global expression analyses and whole genome (or exome) resequencing analyses [14, 54, 71, 72]. Gene-gene interaction and gene-environment interaction are important targets in the genetic analysis of complex diseases. Identification of associated genes will enable the development of gene panels for genetic risk, prognosis, and response to therapy. These approaches have been successfully implemented in studies of other complex diseases such as type 2 diabetes, asthma, and prostate cancer [73–75]. Complex disorders such as CRS can be approached with more powerful molecular technologies, bioinformatics tools and better clinical management.

References

1 Bhattacharyya N: Radiographic stage fails to predict symptom outcomes after endoscopic sinus surgery for chronic rhinosinusitis. Laryngoscope 2006;116:18–22.

2 Orlandi RR, Terrell JE: Analysis of the adult chronic rhinosinusitis working definition. Am J Rhinol 2002;16:7–10.

3 Benson V, Marano MA: Current estimates from the National Health Interview Survey, 1995. Vital Health Stat 10 1998;199:1–428.

4 Adams PF, Hendershot GE, Marano MA: Current estimates from the National Health Interview Survey, 1996. Vital Health Stat 10 1999;200:1–203.

5 Meltzer EO, Hamilos DL, Hadley JA, et al: Rhinosinusitis: establishing definitions for clinical research and patient care. J Allergy Clin Immunol 2004;114 (suppl 6):155–212.

6 Stankiewicz JA, Chow JM: A diagnostic dilemma for chronic rhinosinusitis: definition accuracy and validity. Am J Rhinol 2002;16:199–202.

7 Kaliner MA, Osguthorpe JD, Fireman P, et al: Sinusitis: bench to bedside. Current findings, future directions. J Allergy Clin Immunol 1997;99:S829–S848.

8 Brook I: Sinusitis. Periodontol 2000 2009;49:126–139.

9 Ponikau JU, Sherris DA, Kern EB, et al: The diagnosis and incidence of allergic fungal sinusitis. Mayo Clin Proc 1999;74:877–884.

10 Bhattacharyya N: Air quality influences the prevalence of hay fever and sinusitis. Laryngoscope 2009;119:429–433.

11 Riechelmann H, Deutschle T, Rozsasi A, Keck T, Polzehl D, Burner H: Nasal biomarker profiles in acute and chronic rhinosinusitis. Clin Exp Allergy 2005;35:1186–1191.

12 Cheng YK, Lin CD, Chang WC et al. Increased prevalence of interleukin-1 receptor antagonist gene polymorphism in patients with chronic rhinosinusitis. Arch Otolaryngol Head Neck Surg 2006;132:285–290.

13 Seppanen M, Suvilehto J, Lokki ML, et al: Immunoglobulins and complement factor C4 in adult rhinosinusitis. Clin Exp Immunol 2006;145:219–227.

14 Bosse Y, Bacot F, Montpetit A, et al: Identification of susceptibility genes for complex diseases using pooling-based genome-wide association scans. Hum Genet 2009;125:305–318.

15 Al-Shemari H, Bosse Y, Hudson TJ, et al: Influence of leukotriene gene polymorphisms on chronic rhinosinusitis. BMC Med Genet 2008;9:21.

16 Leigh MW, Pittman JE, Carson JL, et al: Clinical and genetic aspects of primary ciliary dyskinesia/Kartagener syndrome. Genet Med 2009;11:473–487.

17 Babinski D, Trawinska-Bartnicka M: Rhinosinusitis in cystic fibrosis: not a simple story. Int J Pediatr Otorhinolaryngol 2008;72:619–624.

18 Dixon AE: Rhinosinusitis and asthma: the missing link. Curr Opin Pulm Med 2009;15:19–24.

19 Lieu JE, Feinstein AR: Confirmations and surprises in the association of tobacco use with sinusitis. Arch Otolaryngol Head Neck Surg 2000;126:940–946.

20 Briggs RD, Wright ST, Cordes S, Calhoun KH: Smoking in chronic rhinosinusitis: a predictor of poor long-term outcome after endoscopic sinus surgery. Laryngoscope 2004;114:126–128.

21 Bartoloni L, Blouin JL, Pan Y, et al: Mutations in the DNAH11 (axonemal heavy chain dynein type 11) gene cause one form of situs inversus totalis and most likely primary ciliary dyskinesia. Proc Natl Acad Sci USA 2002;99:10282–10286.

22 Sengler C, Lau S, Wahn U, Nickel R: Interactions between genes and environmental factors in asthma and atopy: new developments. Respir Res 2002;3:7.

23 Vercelli D: Advances in asthma and allergy genetics in 2007. J Allergy Clin Immunol 2008;122:267–271.
24 Weiss ST, Raby BA, Rogers A: Asthma genetics and genomics 2009. Curr Opin Genet Dev 2009;19:279–282.
25 Rogers AJ, Raby BA, Lasky-Su JA, et al: Assessing the reproducibility of asthma candidate gene associations, using genome-wide data. Am J Respir Crit Care Med 2009;179:1084–1090.
26 Samter M, Beers RF Jr: Intolerance to aspirin. Clinical studies and consideration of its pathogenesis. Ann Intern Med 1968;68:975–983.
27 Caversaccio M, Hausler R, Helbling A: Otologic manifestations in Samter's syndrome. ORL J Otorhinolaryngol Relat Spec 2009;71:6–10.
28 Fox RW, Lockey RF: The impact of rhinosinusitis on asthma. Curr Allergy Asthma Rep 2003;3:513–518.
29 Ryan MW: Diseases associated with chronic rhinosinusitis: what is the significance? Curr Opin Otolaryngol Head Neck Surg 2008;16:231–236.
30 Agarwal S, Cunningham-Rundles C: Autoimmunity in common variable immunodeficiency. Curr Allergy Asthma Rep 2009;9:347–352.
31 Brandt D, Gershwin ME: Common variable immune deficiency and autoimmunity. Autoimmun Rev 2006;5:465–470.
32 Primary Immunodeficiency Diseases: Report of an IUIS Scientific Committee. International Union of Immunological Societies. Clin Exp Immunol 1999;118(suppl 1):1–28.
33 Eastwood D, Gilmour KC, Nistala K, et al: Prevalence of SAP gene defects in male patients diagnosed with common variable immunodeficiency. Clin Exp Immunol 2004;137:584–588.
34 Moskowitz SM, Chmiel JF, Sternen DL, et al: Clinical practice and genetic counseling for cystic fibrosis and CFTR-related disorders. Genet Med 2008;10: 851–868.
35 Farrell PM, Rosenstein BJ, White TB, et al: Guidelines for diagnosis of cystic fibrosis in newborns through older adults: Cystic Fibrosis Foundation consensus report. J Pediatr 2008;153:S4–S14.
36 Rosenstein BJ, Cutting GR: The diagnosis of cystic fibrosis: a consensus statement. Cystic Fibrosis Foundation Consensus Panel. J Pediatr 1998;132: 589–595.
37 Mickle JE, Cutting GR: Genotype-phenotype relationships in cystic fibrosis. Med Clin North Am 2000;84:597–607.
38 Gu Y, Harley IT, Henderson LB, et al: Identification of IFRD1 as a modifier gene for cystic fibrosis lung disease. Nature 2009;458:1039–1042.
39 Wang X, Moylan B, Leopold DA, et al: Mutation in the gene responsible for cystic fibrosis and predisposition to chronic rhinosinusitis in the general population. JAMA 2000;284:1814–1819.
40 Coste A, Girodon E, Louis S, et al: Atypical sinusitis in adults must lead to looking for cystic fibrosis and primary ciliary dyskinesia. Laryngoscope 2004; 1145:839–843.
41 Leonardi S, Sciuto C, La RM: A missed cystic fibrosis diagnosis in childhood. Allergy Asthma Proc 2005;26:487–488.
42 Noone PG, Knowles MR: 'CFTR-opathies': disease phenotypes associated with cystic fibrosis transmembrane regulator gene mutations. Respir Res 2001; 2:328–332.
43 Miller PW, Hamosh A, Macek M Jr, et al: Cystic fibrosis transmembrane conductance regulator (CFTR) gene mutations in allergic bronchopulmonary aspergillosis. Am J Hum Genet 1996;59:45–51.
44 Wang X, Kim J, McWilliams R, Cutting GR: Increased prevalence of chronic rhinosinusitis in carriers of a cystic fibrosis mutation. Arch Otolaryngol Head Neck Surg 2005;131:237–240.
45 Burger J, Macek M Jr, Stuhrmann M, Reis A, Krawczak M, Schmidtke J: Genetic influences in the formation of nasal polyps. Lancet 1991;337:974.
46 Castellani C, Quinzii C, Altieri S, Mastella G, Assael BM: A pilot survey of cystic fibrosis clinical manifestations in CFTR mutation heterozygotes. Genet Test 2001;5:249–254.
47 Pignatti PF, Bombieri C, Marigo C, Benetazzo M, Luisetti M: Increased incidence of cystic fibrosis gene mutations in adults with disseminated bronchiectasis. Hum Mol Genet 1995;4:635–639.
48 Zariwala MA, Knowles MR, Omran H: Genetic defects in ciliary structure and function. Annu Rev Physiol 2007;69: 423–450.
49 Storm van's GK, Omran H: Primary ciliary dyskinesia: clinical presentation, diagnosis and genetics. Ann Med 2005;37:439–449.
50 Jorissen M, Willems T: The secondary nature of ciliary (dis)orientation in secondary and primary ciliary dyskinesia. Acta Otolaryngol 2004;124:527–531.
51 Geremek M, Zietkiewicz E, Diehl SR, Alizadeh BZ, Wijmenga C, Witt M: Linkage analysis localises a Kartagener syndrome gene to a 3.5 cM region on chromosome 15q24–25. J Med Genet 2006;43:e1.
52 Morillas HN, Zariwala M, Knowles MR: Genetic causes of bronchiectasis: primary ciliary dyskinesia. Respiration 2007;74:252–263.
53 Afzelius BA: Situs inversus and ciliary abnormalities: what is the connection? Int J Dev Biol 1995;39:839–844.
54 Ng SB, Buckingham KJ, Lee C, et al: Exome sequencing identifies the cause of a mendelian disorder. Nat Genet 2009; 42:30–35.
55 Fietta P: Systemic vasculitides: immunogenetics and familial clustering. Clin Exp Rheumatol 2004;22:238–251.
56 Manganelli P, Fietta P, Carotti M, Pesci A, Salaffi F: Respiratory system involvement in systemic vasculitides. Clin Exp Rheumatol 2006;24(2 suppl 41):S48–S59.
57 Gomez-Puerta JA, Hernandez-Rodriguez J, Lopez-Soto A, Bosch X: Antineutrophil cytoplasmic antibody-associated vasculitides and respiratory disease. Chest 2009;136:1101–1111.
58 Brian D: The nasal septum; in Mackay IS, Bull TR (eds): Scott-Brown's Otolaryngology. London, Butterwoth-Heinemann, 1997, pp 4/11/1–4/11/27.
59 Boyce J, Eccles R: Do chronic changes in nasal airflow have any physiological or pathological effect on the nose and paranasal sinuses? A systematic review. Clin Otolaryngol 2006;31:15–19.
60 Stallman JS, Lobo JN, Som PM: The incidence of concha bullosa and its relationship to nasal septal deviation and paranasal sinus disease. AJNR Am J Neuroradiol 2004;25:1613–1618.
61 Harar RP, Chadha NK, Rogers G: The role of septal deviation in adult chronic rhinosinusitis: a study of 500 patients. Rhinology 2004;42:126–130.
62 Earwaker J. Paranasal sinus osteomas: a review of 46 cases. Skeletal Radiol 1993; 22:417–423.
63 McHugh JB, Mukherji SK, Lucas DR: Sino-orbital osteoma: a clinicopathologic study of 45 surgically treated cases with emphasis on tumors with osteoblastoma-like features. Arch Pathol Lab Med 2009;133:1587–1593.

64 Jones K, Korzcak P: The diagnostic significance and management of Gardner's syndrome. Br J Oral Maxillofac Surg 1990;28:80–84.
65 bu-Zeitoon RG, bu-Shahin F, Smalligan RD, Hamati A: Sometimes it's not just sinusitis: nasal type natural killer/T-cell lymphoma. South Med J 2009;102:873–874.
66 Schrijver I: Hereditary non-syndromic sensorineural hearing loss: transforming silence to sound. J Mol Diagn 2004;6:275–284.
67 Welch KO, Marin RS, Pandya A, Arnos KS: Compound heterozygosity for dominant and recessive GJB2 mutations: effect on phenotype and review of the literature. Am J Med Genet A 2007;143A:1567–1573.
68 Cohn ES, Kelley PM: Clinical phenotype and mutations in connexin 26 (DFNB1/GJB2), the most common cause of childhood hearing loss. Am J Med Genet 1999;89:130–136.
69 BuSaba NY, Cunningham MJ: Connexin 26 and 30 genes mutations in patients with chronic rhinosinusitis. Laryngoscope 2008;118:310–313.
70 Costantino M, Lampa E, Nappi G: Effectiveness of sulphur spa therapy with politzer in the treatment of rhinogenic deafness. Acta Otorhinolaryngol Ital 2006;26:7–13.
71 Platt M, Metson R, Stankovic K: Gene-expression signatures of nasal polyps associated with chronic rhinosinusitis and aspirin-sensitive asthma. Curr Opin Allergy Clin Immunol 2009;9:23–28.
72 Stankovic KM, Goldsztein H, Reh DD, Platt MP, Metson R: Gene expression profiling of nasal polyps associated with chronic sinusitis and aspirin-sensitive asthma. Laryngoscope 2008;118:881–889.
73 Prokopenko I, McCarthy MI, Lindgren CM: Type 2 diabetes: new genes, new understanding. Trends Genet 2008;24:613–621.
74 Moffatt MF, Kabesch M, Liang L, et al: Genetic variants regulating ORMDL3 expression contribute to the risk of childhood asthma. Nature 2007;448:470–473.
75 Xu J, Langefeld CD, Zheng SL, et al: Interaction effect of PTEN and CDKN1B chromosomal regions on prostate cancer linkage. Hum Genet 2004;115:255–262.

Xinjing Wang, MD, PhD
National Eye Institute, National Institutes of Health
10 Center Drive, 10D43
Bethesda, MD 20892–1860 (USA)
Tel. +1 301 435 4568, Fax +1 301 451 5499, E-Mail wangx6@mail.nih.gov

Alford RL, Sutton VR (eds): Medical Genetics in the Clinical Practice of ORL.
Adv Otorhinolaryngol. Basel, Karger, 2011, vol 70, pp 122–129

Otosclerosis

Megan Ealy · Richard J.H. Smith

Molecular Otolaryngology Research Laboratories, Department of Otolaryngology, Interdisciplinary Graduate Program in Genetics, University of Iowa, Iowa City, Iowa, USA

Abstract

Otosclerosis is one of the more common forms of adult-onset hearing loss with a prevalence of 0.3–0.4% in Caucasians. It is typically characterized by a conductive hearing loss due to labyrinthine endochondral sclerosis that upon stapedio-vestibular joint invasion results in loss of free motion of the stapes. Its etiology remains poorly understood with both environmental factors and genetic causes implicated in its development. Several environmental influences have been studied and numerous genomic loci have been mapped in families segregating autosomal-dominant otosclerosis. Population-based studies have also identified associations with several genes. These advances are improving our understanding of this complex disease.

Otosclerosis is one of the most common causes of adult-onset hearing loss in the Caucasian population, where it has a prevalence of 0.3–0.4%; its prevalence is lower in blacks, Asians, and Native Americans [1]. The disease is characterized by abnormal bone remodeling in the otic capsule. When lesions of remodeled bone invade the stapedio-vestibular joint, motion of the stapes becomes impaired and a conductive hearing loss results. In addition to conductive hearing loss, about 10% of patients develop sensorineural hearing loss [2, 3]. Although the cause of the sensorineural component is unknown, it may be related to remodeling of the bony labyrinth immediately surrounding the cochlea, a process that releases enzymes which can damage the cochlea.

Clinically, otosclerosis is a progressive conductive hearing loss with an average age of onset in the 30s. It occurs bilaterally in 70–80% of the cases and in addition to hearing loss, nearly half of the patients report tinnitus; 10% of patients also experience vertigo [4, 5]. The female:male prevalence is 1.5–2:1 [6]. Histological otosclerosis is far more common, occurring in up to 12% of the Caucasian population. It does not lead to a hearing loss phenotype as it is detectable only by temporal bone analysis at autopsy (or occasionally by high-resolution computed tomography) [7]. Interestingly, there is no gender bias noted in studies of histological otosclerosis.

Treatment of otosclerosis consists of stapes microsurgery to correct the effects of the conductive hearing loss. The procedure, a stapedotomy, involves the removal of the suprastructure of the stapes followed by opening part of the stapes footplate with a microdrill or laser. A prosthesis is fitted into the opening made in the footplate, connecting the incus to the oval window and restoring ossicular conduction by bypassing the fixed footplate [8, 9]. The surgery is generally very successful although some individuals have to undergo revision surgery (which is less successful) [2, 3]. There is no treatment for the sensorineural component of the disease; however, cochlear implantation for individuals with profound hearing loss due to otosclerosis has been effective [10–12].

In spite of numerous studies looking at environmental and genetic factors, our understanding of the pathophysiology of otosclerosis remains limited. Viral infection and hormones have been implicated; however, the obvious ethnic bias suggests that genetic components play a major role in disease pathogenesis. Additional evidence to support the role of genetics includes familial inheritance studies that to date have identified eight different otosclerosis loci *(OTSC1–8)*. Population-based case-control studies have also associated a number of genes with otosclerosis.

Bone Remodeling and the Otic Capsule

Bone remodeling is a dynamic process coordinated by osteoclasts (bone resorbing cells) and osteoblasts (bone-forming cells) [13, 14]. Osteoclasts differentiate from the hematopoietic cell lineage [15]. Their maturation requires the presence of the RANK ligand (RANKL), which is produced by osteoblasts. Once RANKL is bound by the receptor RANK on the monocyte precursor, osteoclast differentiation begins [16]. Mature active osteoclasts are giant multinucleated cells that have a polarity and a ruffled border that secretes the lysosomal enzymes required for bone resorption [17]. As old bone is resorbed, new bone matrix is deposited by osteoblasts, which differentiate from mesenchymal stem cells in the presence of osteogenic proteins such as the bone morphogenetic proteins [18].

The human skeleton undergoes bone turnover at a rate of about 10% per year, however the otic capsule undergoes very little to no remodeling. In regions surrounding the perilymph spaces, for example, the otic capsule turns over at the incredibly slow rate of 0.13% per year [19]. Decreased remodeling is due to the production of osteoprogerin (OPG) by the cochlea. This RANKL antagonist travels through a network of canaliculi in the otic capsule to maintain the static state of otic capsule bone [20, 21]. In Opg –/– mice, the absence of osteoprotegerin leads to bone remodeling in the otic capsule and a conductive hearing loss due to fixation of the stapes [21].

The otic capsule develops through a process of endochondral ossification. Endochondral bone is formed through a cartilage intermediate, which becomes calcified as it matures. In the otic capsule, embryonic cartilaginous remnants persist even into adulthood and are known as globuli interossei [22]. The otic capsule also contains inactive bone cells such as osteocytes, which are terminally differentiated osteoblasts that maintain the mineralization of the bone.

Otosclerosis occurs in phases with the first phase being one of active remodeling, also called the otospongiotic phase [23]. This phase is characterized by activated osteoclasts and is highly vascularized. The second phase is heralded by new bone deposition by osteoblasts, which can then be mineralized; the final phase involves replacement by fibrous tissue [23]. Determining the triggers of the otospongiotic stage of otosclerosis is believed to be key to developing new treatments for the disease.

Environmental Factors and Otosclerosis

A variety of environmental factors have been considered in the development of otosclerosis. One hypothesis, for example, states that persistent measles virus infection may have a role in otosclerosis. In support of this possibility, several groups have found evidence of measles virus in otosclerotic lesions using a number of molecular techniques [24–27]. However, whether viral infection acts as a trigger for the onset of disease remains to be shown. A decline in the incidence of otosclerosis has been reported and attributed to the introduction of the measles vaccine [28]. However, the vaccine has only been available for the last 40 years, and many of those vaccinated have not reached the average age of disease onset to draw definite conclusions. The apparent gender bias in clinical otosclerosis has also prompted work on different hormones and some studies suggest that estrogen may have a role in disease [5], but studies of disease progression during pregnancy have yielded conflicting results [29, 30].

Genetics of Otosclerosis

The obvious ethnic bias of otosclerosis speaks for the importance of a genetic background. In fact, early studies of otosclerosis noted the autosomal-dominant inheritance pattern with reduced penetrance [30–32]. A number of other inheritance patterns were also described including digenic inheritance and an even more complicated X-linked dominant–autosomal-recessive inheritance pattern [33, 34]. Today, otosclerosis is generally considered an autosomal-dominant disease with reduced penetrance; however, half of all the cases are sporadic [35].

Family Linkage Studies

Family-based linkage studies have led to the mapping of eight different *OTSC* loci although no disease-causing mutations have been identified in any of these mapped families. Some of the best candidate genes in each region have been screened, but a great number of genes remain to be screened. Since many of the best candidates for bone remodeling are also expressed in many other tissues, and since there are distinct differences between the otic capsule and the skeletal bone remodeling, regulatory elements may play an important role [36–42].

Recently, the likely causative gene for otosclerosis has been identified in a Belgian *OTSC2* family. The *OTSC2* locus maps to chromosome 7q34–36 and includes the T cell receptor locus [42]. Analysis of T cells in this family has shown that there is an increased population of $CD28^{null}$ cells in patients, suggesting disturbed T cell development and aging. *OTSC2* patients also have decreased levels of TCRβ mRNA and lower percentage of circulating $TCR\alpha\beta^{+}$ T cells as compared to controls [43]. These findings are consistent with a change in regulation of the *TCRB* gene and implicate the TRB locus as the *OTSC2* gene although a genetic variant linked to the *TCRB* gene in *OTSC2* patients remains to be identified.

The story of *OTSC2* shows that coding variation may not be involved in disease onset. For example, the *OTSC1* locus is located on 15q25-q26 and no coding mutation in any of the known genes in this interval has been found. The interval does include aggrecan *(ACAN)* and just outside the interval is *FURIN*, a gene encoding furin, which has a known function in bone remodeling [40]. Furin cleaves members of the TGFβ superfamily of molecules to produce the mature forms of these proteins. Perhaps a regulatory element for this gene resides within the linked region, and variation in this potential element leads to altered expression in *OTSC1* patients. Screening of evolutionarily conserved elements that are predicted to contain transcription factor binding sites would be a next good step in identifying the disease causing mutation in this family.

OTSC3 was mapped in a large Cypriot family to the MHC locus on chromosome 6 [38]. Previous studies on the HLA antigens have shown an increase in HLA-A11, Bw35, and B14 in Greek individuals with a family history of otosclerosis [44]. Perhaps a similar analysis of the HLA proteins in serum from family members will be helpful in determining what is causing disease in this family. However, if one or more the HLA proteins are involved in this family's disease, it will be interesting to determine how these play a role in bone remodeling. Whether these genes have some sort of capacity for controlling lineage fate of osteoblast or osteoclast precursors would need to be determined.

Similar scenarios should be considered upon reanalysis of the remaining *OTSC* families. With next-generation sequencing, deep sequencing can be used to identify disease-causing variation at these loci by studying functional elements like promoters and enhancers, 5′ and 3′ UTRs, and intronic sequence, as well as coding exons. In addition to nucleotide variation, differences in structural variation including copy number variation, insertions and deletions can be considered.

Candidate Gene Association Studies

A number of population-based candidate gene studies have identified associations with *COL1A1*, *TGFB1*, *BMP2*, *BMP4*, *AGT*, and *ACE* and otosclerosis; however, the associations with *COL1A1*, *AGT*, and *ACE* are controversial [45, 46]. The association with *COL1A1* was first demonstrated in an American otosclerosis population [47]. A stronger association of the Sp1-binding site polymorphism in the first intron of *COL1A1* was later demonstrated in a comparison of 100 otosclerosis patients to unmatched controls [48]. Another study identified haplotypes including a single nucleotide polymorphism in an Sp1 transcription factor binding site that are associated with otosclerosis in American and German groups [49]. It was shown that these polymorphisms affect binding of transcription factors, and it is hypothesized that increased homotrimers of COL1A1 contribute to abnormal bone deposition in the otic capsule. Consistent with this possibility, in the mouse with a targeted deletion of *COL1A2*, the stapes footplate is thicker and there is a mild hearing loss. While association has been shown with this gene in two separate American populations and a German population, an attempt to replicate association with *COL1A1* in a Spanish population was unable to confirm an association with *COL1A1* [45].

The second association with otosclerosis was shown in a two separate populations. The T263I coding variant in the gene, *TGFB1*, is associated with otosclerosis in both Belgian-Dutch and French populations [50]. Functional analysis of this variant showed that the I263 allele induces transcription of a TGF-β1-responsive reporter gene to a higher level than the T263 allele. The I263 allele is predicted to be protective since it is over-represented in the controls in both the Belgian and French populations. An overactive form of TGF-β1 may limit the otospongiotic phase of otosclerosis if osteoclastogenesis is inhibited. More work will be needed to determine how this variant protects against disease.

Genetic associations with two additional members of the TGFβ superfamily, *BMP2* and *BMP4*, have been associated with otosclerosis in the same populations used to detect the *TGFB1* association [51]. Both *BMP2* and *BMP4* are expressed in otosclerotic lesions and with *BMP7* have roles in otic capsule development [52–54]. The associated SNP in *BMP2* may play a role in gene regulation as it is located in the 3′UTR of the gene, while the associated SNP in *BMP4* is a coding variant A152V.

In an attempt to explain the female disease bias, a study has shown association with genes in the renin-angiotensin-aldosterone system and otosclerosis [55]. These genes were considered as candidates because they are upregulated during pregnancy [56]. However, studies investigating the effect of pregnancy on hearing loss caused by otosclerosis have been performed with conflicting results [29, 30]. The association shown with polymorphisms in *AGT* and *ACE* in a French otosclerosis population have not been replicated in two other populations – a Belgian-Dutch population and a separate French population [46].

A truly associated allele that confers a major effect on the disease would be expected to be associated across multiple test groups [57]. The ability to replicate association results is therefore very important and depends on appropriate study design with careful consideration of sample size, population substructure and control selection. Association studies are normally performed using markers (in most cases SNPs) that are highly prevalent in a population, many of which are unlikely to be the causative variant in the disease but rather linked to the causative gene [58]. Since small differences in linkage disequilibrium (LD) structure across populations can differ slightly, it is wise to consider typing several markers in the gene when trying to replicate gene-disease associations [57].

Once an association with a gene is found, work must be done to identify causative variants in the gene. Since associations are conducted with common variants in the genome, these are most likely not the causative variants in the gene. Deep resequencing of the gene should be conducted to determine what variation is present in the gene [59]. For the *TGFB1* association, screening of otosclerosis patients has found several variants within this gene that are not present in controls. Sequence analysis of *TGFB1* in the Belgian-Dutch and French populations yielded three rare nonsynonymous mutations [60]. Two different variants at the cleavage site for the signal peptide of TGF-β1 were found. The first, a G29E variant, was detected in two Belgian-Dutch otosclerosis patients, and is predicted to alter cleavage of the signal peptide. The second, a G29A variant, was found in a French patient. This variant is not predicted to affect cleavage according to in silico analysis; however, it potentially eliminates an N-myristolation site on this residue. A third variant, T241I, was identified in a Belgian-Dutch individual and may change a predicted phosphorylation or amidation site in the latency associated peptide domain of TGF-β1. Based on the hypothesis that the I263 identified in the original association study is a protective variant that increases TGF-β1 activity, it would be expected that these three rare variants found in otosclerosis patients would have the opposite effect on TGF-β1 function. However, functional analyses of these variants are needed to determine relevance to disease.

Once variants have been found, functional testing should be done to understand how these variants lead to disease. The precise tests will depend on the gene of interest. For example, TGF-β1 is a known regulator of bone remodeling and studies focused on osteoblast and osteoclast differentiation, maturation, and function are needed.

Genome-Wide Association Study

A genome-wide association study (GWAS) offers a hypothesis-free approach to identify genes involved in otosclerosis, and to date, one such study has been completed. The original association using a pooled GWAS design identified the gene encoding reelin as an important factor in otosclerosis; results were then confirmed in multiple different populations [61, 62]. Reelin is an extracellular matrix protein important in neuronal positioning during brain development [63]. Although not previously considered 'interesting' in otosclerosis, based on the GWAS data, expression studies have been completed and show that *RELN* mRNA is present in human stapes samples and Reln protein is present in mouse inner ear. A recent study looking at differential gene expression in osteocytes and osteoblasts in mice has also shown that Reln is expressed to a higher degree in osteocytes than osteoblasts [64]. This difference is relevant to otosclerosis since osteocytes are found within the globuli interossei. How Reelin promotes bone remodeling will provide insight into otosclerosis and possibly other diseases of bone metabolism.

Gene Expression in Otosclerosis

To complement genetic studies, several expression studies have been performed. Analysis of different bone metabolism proteins has shown expression of bone morphogenetic proteins in otosclerotic lesions [52]. Expression of several proteins involved in measles virus infection has also been described [25, 27, 65], and a genome-wide expression study has been conducted [66].

Expression studies enable us to organize our understanding at the molecular level by identifying important systems and pathways in otosclerosis. In addition to the presence and absence of particular proteins, it is also important to know what splice variants are present in diseased versus healthy tissue. It is predicted that around 90% of genes are alternatively spliced and it is highly likely that differences in splicing contribute to disease development [67]. As an example, work looking at splice variants of the measles virus receptor CD46 has identified a number of otosclerosis-specific splice variants of this gene [68]. As with the advancement of sequencing technologies for genetic screening, technologies for the analysis of alternative splicing continue to improve. Tiled exon arrays are available that can be used to predict alternative splicing in tissue samples. Deep resequencing of RNA molecules is also possible using next-generation sequencing technology. These techniques are both quantitative and qualitative and will be an important part of future studies.

Concluding Remarks

Much work has been done to identify environmental and genetic factors that contribute to otosclerosis. Work on both familial and sporadic cases has led to a compilation of data that underscores the complexity of the disease. By identifying specific triggers and clarifying the genetics of otosclerosis, we will be better able to tailor treatments that complement and hopefully lessen the need for stapes surgery.

References

1 Declau F, et al: Prevalence of otosclerosis in an unselected series of temporal bones. Otol Neurotol 2001;22:596–602.
2 Browning GG, Gatehouse S: Sensorineural hearing loss in stapedial otosclerosis. Ann Otol Rhinol Laryngol 1984;93:13–16.
3 Ramsay HA, Linthicum FH Jr: Mixed hearing loss in otosclerosis: indication for long-term follow-up. Am J Otol 1994; 15:536–539.
4 Gristwood RE, Venables WN: Otosclerosis and chronic tinnitus. Ann Otol Rhinol Laryngol 2003;112:398–403.
5 Menger DJ, Tange RA: The aetiology of otosclerosis: a review of the literature. Clin Otolaryngol Allied Sci 2003;28:112–120.
6 Gordon MA: The genetics of otosclerosis: a review. Am J Otol 1989;10:426–438.
7 Declau F, et al: Prevalence of histologic otosclerosis: an unbiased temporal bone study in Caucasians. Adv Otorhinolaryngol 2007;65:6–16.
8 Fisch U: Stapedotomy versus stapedectomy. Am J Otol 1982;4:112–117.
9 Gantz BJ, et al: Argon laser stapedotomy. Ann Otol Rhinol Laryngol 1982;91:25–26.
10 Mosnier I, et al: Cochlear implantation and far-advanced otosclerosis. Adv Otorhinolaryngol 2007;65:323–327.
11 Psillas G, et al: Far-advanced otosclerosis and cochlear implantation. B-Ent 2007; 3:67–71.
12 Ruckenstein MJ, et al: Management of far advanced otosclerosis in the era of cochlear implantation. Otol Neurotol 2001;22:471–474.
13 Petrtyl M, Hert J, Fiala P: Spatial organization of the haversian bone in man. J Biomech 1996;29:161–169.
14 Parfitt AM: Osteonal and hemi-osteonal remodeling: the spatial and temporal framework for signal traffic in adult human bone. J Cell Biochem 1994;55: 273–286.
15 Teitelbaum SL: Bone resorption by osteoclasts. Science 2000;289:1504–1508.
16 Hadjidakis DJ, Androulakis II: Bone remodeling. Ann NY Acad Sci 2006; 1092:385–396.
17 Vaananen HK, et al: The cell biology of osteoclast function. J Cell Sci 2000; 113:377–381.
18 Bianco P, et al: Bone marrow stromal stem cells: nature, biology, and potential applications. Stem Cells 2001;19:180–192.
19 Frisch T, et al: Estimation of volume referent bone turnover in the otic capsule after sequential point labeling. Ann Otol Rhinol Laryngol 2000;109:33–39.

20 Zehnder AF, et al: Osteoprotegerin in the inner ear may inhibit bone remodeling in the otic capsule. Laryngoscope 2005;115:172–177.
21 Zehnder AF, et al: Osteoprotegrin knockout mice demonstrate abnormal remodeling of the otic capsule and progressive hearing loss. Laryngoscope 2006;116:201–206.
22 Schuknecht HF: Pathology of the Ear, ed 2. Philadelphia, Lea & Febiger, 1993.
23 Niedermeyer HP, Arnold W: Etiopathogenesis of otosclerosis. ORL J Otorhinolaryngol Relat Spec 2002;64:114–119.
24 Arnold W, Friedmann I: Detection of measles and rubella-specific antigens in the endochondral ossification zone in otosclerosis. Laryngol Rhinol Otol (Stuttg) 1987;66:167–171.
25 McKenna MJ, Mills BG: Ultrastructural and immunohistochemical evidence of measles virus in active otosclerosis. Acta Otolaryngol Suppl 1990;470:130–139; discussion 139–140.
26 Karosi T, et al: Measles virus prevalence in otosclerotic stapes footplate samples. Otol Neurotol 2004;25:451–456.
27 Niedermeyer H, et al: Evidence of measles virus RNA in otosclerotic tissue. ORL J Otorhinolaryngol Relat Spec 1994;56:130–132.
28 Arnold W: Some remarks on the histopathology of otosclerosis. Adv Otorhinolaryngol 2007;65:25–30.
29 Lippy WH, et al: Does pregnancy affect otosclerosis? Laryngoscope 2005;115:1833–1836.
30 Morrison AW: Genetic factors in otosclerosis. Ann R Coll Surg Engl 1967;41:202–237.
31 Albrecht W: Ueber der Vererbung der hereditären Labyrinth-schwerhörigkeit und der Otosclerose. Arch Ohrenheilk Nas Kehlkopfheilk 1922;110:15–48.
32 Larsson A: Otosclerosis: a genetic and clinical study. Acta Otolaryngol Suppl 1960;154:1–86.
33 Bauer J, Stein C: Vererbung und Konstitution bei Ohrenkrankheiten. Z Konstitutionslehre 1925;10:483–545.
34 Hernandez-Orozco F, Courtney GT: Genetic aspects of clinical otosclerosis. Ann Otol Rhinol Laryngol 1964;73:632–644.
35 Cawthorn T: Otosclerosis. J Laryngol Otol 1955;69:437–456.
36 Bel Hadj Ali I, et al: A new locus for otosclerosis, OTSC8, maps to the pericentromeric region of chromosome 9. Hum Genet 2008;123:267–272.
37 Brownstein Z, et al: Chromosomal mapping and phenotypic characterization of hereditary otosclerosis linked to the OTSC4 locus. Arch Otolaryngol Head Neck Surg 2006;132:416–424.
38 Chen W, et al: Linkage of otosclerosis to a third locus (OTSC3) on human chromosome 6p21.3–22.3. J Med Genet 2002;39:473–477.
39 Thys M, et al: A seventh locus for otosclerosis, OTSC7, maps to chromosome 6q13–16.1. Eur J Hum Genet 2007;15:362–368.
40 Tomek MS, et al: Localization of a gene for otosclerosis to chromosome 15q25-q26. Hum Mol Genet 1998;7:285–290.
41 Van Den Bogaert K, et al: A fifth locus for otosclerosis, OTSC5, maps to chromosome 3q22–24. J Med Genet 2004;41:450–453.
42 Van Den Bogaert K, et al: A second gene for otosclerosis, OTSC2, maps to chromosome 7q34–36. Am J Hum Genet 2001;68:495–500.
43 Schrauwen I, et al: Involvement of T-cell receptor-beta alterations in the development of otosclerosis linked to OTSC2. Genes Immun 2010;11:246–253.
44 Gregoriadis S, et al: HLA antigens and otosclerosis: a possible new genetic factor. Arch Otolaryngol 1982;108:769–771.
45 Rodriguez L, et al: Proposed association between the COL1A1 and COL1A2 genes and otosclerosis is not supported by a case-control study in Spain. Am J Med Genet A 2004;128:19–22.
46 Schrauwen I, et al: No evidence for association between the renin-angiotensin-aldosterone system and otosclerosis in a large Belgian-Dutch population. Otol Neurotol 2009;30:1079–1083.
47 McKenna MJ, et al: Association of COL1A1 and otosclerosis: evidence for a shared genetic etiology with mild osteogenesis imperfecta. Am J Otol 1998;19:604–610.
48 McKenna MJ, Nguyen-Huynh AT, Kristiansen AG: Association of otosclerosis with Sp1 binding site polymorphism in COL1A1 gene: evidence for a shared genetic etiology with osteoporosis. Otol Neurotol 2004;25:447–450.
49 Chen W, et al: Single-nucleotide polymorphisms in the COL1A1 regulatory regions are associated with otosclerosis. Clin Genet 2007;71:406–414.
50 Thys M, et al: The coding polymorphism T263I in TGF-beta1 is associated with otosclerosis in two independent populations. Hum Mol Genet 2007;16:2021–2030.
51 Schrauwen I, et al: Association of bone morphogenetic proteins with otosclerosis. J Bone Miner Res 2008;23:507–516.
52 Lehnerdt G, et al: Immunohistochemical evidence of BMP-2, -4 and -7 activity in otospongiosis. Acta Otolaryngol 2007;128:1–5.
53 Frenz DA, Liu W, Capparelli M: Role of BMP-2a in otic capsule chondrogenesis. Ann NY Acad Sci 1996;785:256–258.
54 Liu W, et al: Bone morphogenetic protein 4 (BMP4): a regulator of capsule chondrogenesis in the developing mouse inner ear. Dev Dyn 2003;226:427–438.
55 Imauchi Y, et al: Relation between renin-angiotensin-aldosterone system and otosclerosis: a genetic association and in vitro study. Otol Neurotol 2008;29:295–301.
56 Schrier RW, Durr JA: Pregnancy: an overfill or underfill state. Am J Kidney Dis 1987;9:284–289.
57 Tabor HK, Risch NJ, Myers RM: Candidate-gene approaches for studying complex genetic traits: practical considerations. Nat Rev Genet 2002;3:391–397.
58 Syvanen AC: Accessing genetic variation: genotyping single nucleotide polymorphisms. Nat Rev Genet 2001;2:930–942.
59 Li B, Leal SM: Methods for detecting associations with rare variants for common diseases: application to analysis of sequence data. Am J Hum Genet 2008;83:311–321.
60 Thys M, et al: Detection of rare nonsynonymous variants in TGFB1 in otosclerosis patients. Ann Hum Genet 2009;73:171–175.
61 Schrauwen I, et al: Genetic variants in the RELN gene are associated with otosclerosis in different European populations. Hum Genet, Accepted for publication.
62 Schrauwen I, et al: Genetic variants in the RELN gene are associated with otosclerosis in multiple European populations. Hum Genet 2010;127:155–162.
63 Quattrocchi CC, et al: Reelin is a serine protease of the extracellular matrix. J Biol Chem 2002;277:303–309.

64 Paic F, et al: Identification of differentially expressed genes between osteoblasts and osteocytes. Bone 2009;45:682–692.
65 Karosi T, et al: Codetection of measles virus and tumor necrosis factor-alpha mRNA in otosclerotic stapes footplates. Laryngoscope 2005;115:1291–1297.
66 Ealy M, et al: Gene expression analysis of human otosclerotic stapedial footplates. Hear Res 2008;240:80–86.
67 Wang ET, et al: Alternative isoform regulation in human tissue transcriptomes. Nature 2008;456:470–476.
68 Karosi T, et al: Disease-associated novel CD46 splicing variants and pathologic bone remodeling in otosclerosis. Laryngoscope 2008;118:669–676.

Richard J.H. Smith
Pediatrics and Internal Medicine – Division of Nephrology, The University of Iowa
200 Hawkins Drive – 21151 PFP
Iowa City, IA 52242 (USA)
Tel. +1 319 356 3612, Fax +1 319 356 4108, E-Mail richard-smith@uiowa.edu

Alford RL, Sutton VR (eds): Medical Genetics in the Clinical Practice of ORL.
Adv Otorhinolaryngol. Basel, Karger, 2011, vol 70, pp 130–134

Genetics of Vestibulopathies

Joanna C. Jen

Department of Neurology, UCLA School of Medicine, Los Angeles, Calif., USA

Abstract

This review focuses on recent advances in the genetics of familial vestibular disorders including benign recurrent vertigo, bilateral vestibulopathy, and familial Meniere's disease. To date, no genetic causes have been identified in these vestibular conditions. This limited progress has been attributed to the subtle phenotypes, requirement for sophisticated vestibular testing, likely complex nature of these conditions, lack of animal models and reliance on patient history with a paucity of objective diagnostic criteria. Studying vestibular disorders in carefully characterized multiplex families will provide us genetic clues to expand our knowledge of vestibular development, degeneration, structure and function to help us improve the diagnosis and develop effective treatment of vestibulopathies.

Several neurotological conditions causing recurrent episodes of vertigo variably associated with progressive impairment of vestibular function have long been recognized to occur in families and therefore may have a genetic basis: benign recurrent vertigo, bilateral vestibulopathy, and familial Meniere's disease. In contrast to much recent advancement in identifying the genetic basis of deafness (as discussed in several chapters in this book), research on vestibular disorders has lagged behind, with no genetic cause identified in humans to date. This lack of progress has been attributed to the subtle phenotypes that require sophisticated vestibular testing using quantitative rotational stimuli available only at major academic centers, which further hampers the identification of kindreds for genetic studies. Just as the study of hereditary hearing loss has greatly enhanced our understanding of the role of the cochlea in hearing, studying inherited vestibular disorders will expand our knowledge of vestibular development, structure and function to help us diagnose and develop effective treatment for vestibulopathies. Collaborative efforts will facilitate the establishment of diagnostic criteria, which are critically important for patient identification and recruitment for studies in clinical characterization and genetic investigation and for potential clinical trials in the future.

Benign Recurrent Vertigo

Clinical Features

Benign recurrent vertigo (BRV) is a common disorder affecting up to 2% of the adult population [1]. Many families have multiple affected members, suggesting familial transmission. This disorder is termed benign because it is not associated with an identifiable cause or neurological sign. It is also known as benign paroxysmal vertigo of childhood [2] and BRV of adulthood [3]. Furthermore, many patients with BRV suffer from migraine such that terms including vestibular migraine [4], migrainous vertigo [5, 6] or migraine-associated vertigo [7] have also been proposed. Excluded from BRV is benign paroxysmal positional vertigo, which is caused by canalolithiasis and cupulolithiasis [8].

Basser [2] described an episodic disorder that he called benign paroxysmal vertigo in otherwise completely normal children who suddenly became frightened and staggered, as though drunk, and exhibited pallor, diaphoresis and often vomiting. Some children reported a true spinning sensation. The spells typically lasted for several minutes. The children then were usually able to return to play without any untoward effects. These recurrent vertigo spells usually begin early and can recur throughout childhood, either spontaneously remitting or persisting into adulthood. Benign paroxysmal vertigo of childhood has subsequently been shown in numerous studies to be strongly associated with migraine [9–15] such that it is considered a childhood periodic syndrome that is a precursor of migraine in the Classification of Headache Disorders defined by the International Headache Society.

Slater [3] described a series of patients who experienced recurrent episodes of vertigo with nausea and vomiting, usually beginning in adulthood, which he called benign recurrent vertigo (BRV). The attacks often occurred on awakening in the morning, being particularly prominent in women around the time of their menstrual period. Duration varied from a few minutes to as long as 3–4 days, and patients were asymptomatic between spells. During the episodes, there were no auditory symptoms, specifically no hearing loss, tinnitus or ear fullness. Many patients either had migraine themselves or a family history of migraine. The episodes of vertigo have several features in common with migraine including precipitation by alcohol, lack of sleep, stress, and increased prevalence in women. The temporal concurrence of benign recurrent vertigo and migraine has been reported to be between 30 and 70% in various studies [4, 7, 16–18]. Whether and how benign recurrent vertigo may be related mechanistically to migraine remains controversial.

Genetics

In an initial effort to genetically define BRV, genetic linkage mapping was performed on twenty multigenerational families [19]. There was suggestive linkage to chromosome 22q12, with evidence of heterogeneity. Of note, BRV and migraine did not appear to be allelic in these families. The determination of causative alleles in BRV awaits additional family- and population-based linkage and association studies. Clear definition of the clinical features may allow stratification and enrichment of subgroups within BRV to facilitate gene or association allele identification.

Bilateral Vestibulopathy

Clinical Features

Bilateral vestibulopathy results from impaired function of both peripheral labyrinths, leading to impaired vestibule-ocular reflex and thus an inability to stabilize gaze with rapid head movement. Patients typically first notice brief episodes of vertigo in the second or third decade, then followed years later by imbalance and head movement-dependent oscillopsia. There are no associated hearing changes or baseline hearing impairment; audiometric findings are consistently normal. The gain by quantitative rotational testing is greater than 2 SDs below the normal mean for both sinusoidal (0.05 Hz, 120°/s) and step (120°/s, $140°/s^2$) changes in angular velocity. Patients with bilateral vestibulopathy typically do not have other neurological deficits, but there are rare patients with cerebellar ataxia or peripheral neuropathy [20–22].

Patient history is generally incompatible with viral, vascular or autoimmune etiology; it is also negative for trauma or exposure to ototoxic antibiotics. In a recent retrospective study of bilateral vestibulopathy, a likely cause was identified in less than half of the patients, emphasizing the challenge in the diagnosis as well as the limitations in our understanding of the mechanisms underlying bilateral vestibulopathy [22]. Of interest, most patients with bilateral vestibulopathy also meet the International Headache Society (IHS; 2004) criteria for migraine with or without aura. It is unclear whether migraine and vestibulopathy are related, since migraine is highly prevalent and is often observed in relatives without vestibulopathy.

Clinically, the effects of bilateral vestibulopathy are often subtle and affected patients may not even be aware of them. Some patients will have episodes of vertigo but others will have only mild imbalance and visual distortion due to oscillopsia. If the bilateral vestibular loss occurs early in life, it may be compensated for without ever causing significant symptoms. The loss of vestibular function is compensated for by other sensory systems, particularly somatosensation and vision. By contrast, hearing loss, even to a mild degree, is readily apparent to the patient and so hearing loss families are much more readily identified. Even though symptoms of bilateral vestibulopathy can be subtle in some family members, in others they can be more disabling. If patients with bilateral vestibulopathy lose vision or peripheral sensation due to peripheral neuropathy, the combination of sensory loss with vestibulopathy can be devastating [21].

Genetics

A handful of families with bilateral vestibulopathy and migraine spanning several generations have been described [23], as was a small family with vestibulopathy without migraine [24]. Verhagen et al. [25] described two brothers and a sister with bilateral vestibular loss and normal hearing, apparently inherited on an autosomal recessive basis, since the mother and father each had large families and none described any symptoms suggesting vestibular loss. The symptoms in the three patients began in infancy and may even have been present at birth. None of the affected patients complained of vertigo attacks.

In contrast to the ever-increasing number of deafness genes, no mutations have been identified in bilateral vestibulopathy with normal hearing. Analogous to nonsyndromic inherited deafness, bilateral vestibulopathy may be a monogenic disorder with different modes of inheritance, including autosomal dominant, autosomal recessive, sex-linked or mitochondrial. There has been a single report of linkage analysis in families with a dominantly inherited bilateral vestibulopathy syndrome associated with migraine and normal hearing [26]. The disease loci in four families with bilateral vestibulopathy and migraine demonstrated suggestive linkage to a 34-cM region on chromosome 6q. Different haplotypes were found in these families, suggesting distinct genetic background and origin. The small family with vestibulopathy but not migraine did not map to the same region, further suggesting genetic heterogeneity. There is continuing effort to identify patients with idiopathic bilateral vestibulopathy.

Meniere's Disease

Clinical Features

Meniere's disease is characterized by episodic and recurrent vertigo, fluctuating low-frequency hearing loss, tinnitus, and aural pressure [27]. Only a small number of patients with recurrent episodic vertigo have associated auditory symptoms that meet the diagnostic criteria for Meniere's disease. Recurrent episodic vertigo with hearing impairment is rarely seen in multiple members in the same family.

The causes underlying Meniere's disease remain unknown. The association between Meniere's disease and autoimmune disorders has led some to hypothesize an immune-mediated disease process. Meniere's disease is mostly sporadic, and no monozygotic twins with Meniere's disease have been described. There have been rare reports on familial Meniere's disease [28–35]. The transmission of Meniere's disease in the majority of these families was most consistent with an autosomal dominant mode of inheritance, but recessive transmission in one of the reported families has also been proposed. The high prevalence of migraine in patients with Meniere's disease has long been recognized; whether and how migraine may damage the inner ear to cause Meniere's disease remains controversial [34, 36, 37].

Genetics

Of the approximately 40 dominantly inherited hearing loss syndromes (DFNA), only 2 are associated with vestibulopathy: DFNA9 with mutations in the *COCH* gene [38], and DFNA 11 with mutations in the *MYO7* gene [39]. In one series, more than 25% of patients with DFNA9 met the clinical diagnostic criteria for Meniere's disease [40]. Although *COCH* mutations are important causes of autosomal dominant hearing impairment with vestibular dysfunction, they appear to contribute little to sporadic Meniere's disease when further investigated in large series of sporadic Meniere's disease [41, 42].

Attempts at linkage mapping by various groups concur that there is genetic heterogeneity, which is not unexpected, as is the case for inherited deafness syndromes. Initial analysis demonstrated positive linkage to chromosome 14 in four families with Meniere's disease [33]. The disease locus for a large Swedish family with Meniere's disease spanning five generations [30] was previously mapped to chromosome 12p12.3 [43]. The identification of another small kindred with Meniere's disease with a shared haplotype suggested common ancestral origin for the two kindreds to further narrow the candidate region. Recent haplotype analysis using microsatellite markers on chromosome 12p in an additional 15 Swedish families with at least two members affected by Meniere's disease demonstrated suggestive allelic association of markers on chromosome 12p, suggesting a possible ancestral haplotype for familial Meniere's disease in Sweden [44]. However, direct sequencing of several genes in the candidate region, including *PIK3C2G*, *RERGL*, and U2 small nuclear RNA, has not revealed any sequence variation that may be pathogenic.

References

1 Oh AK, Lee H, Jen JC, Corona S, Jacobson KM, Baloh RW: Familial benign recurrent vertigo. Am J Med Genet 2001;100:287–291.

2 Basser LS: Benign paroxysmal vertigo of childhood: a variety of vestibular neuronitis. Brain 1964;87:141–152.

3 Slater R: Benign recurrent vertigo. J Neurol Neurosurg Psychiatry 1979;42: 363–367.

4 Dieterich M, Brandt T: Episodic vertigo related to migraine (90 cases): vestibular migraine? J Neurol 1999;246:883–892.

5 Neuhauser H, Leopold M, von Brevern M, Arnold G, Lempert T: The interrelations of migraine, vertigo, and migrainous vertigo. Neurology 2001;56:436–441.

6 Neuhauser HK, Radtke A, von Brevern M, Feldmann M, Lezius F, Ziese T, Lempert T: Migrainous vertigo: prevalence and impact on quality of life. Neurology 2006;67:1028–1033.

7 Cutrer FM, Baloh RW: Migraine-associated dizziness. Headache 1992;32: 300–304.

8 Fife TD, Iverson DJ, Lempert T, Furman JM, Baloh RW, Tusa RJ, Hain TC, Herdman S, Morrow MJ, Gronseth GS: Practice parameter: therapies for benign paroxysmal positional vertigo (an evidence-based review): report of the Quality Standards Subcommittee of the American Academy of Neurology. Neurology 2008;70:2067–2074.

9 Fenichel GM: Migraine as a cause of benign paroxysmal vertigo of childhood. J Pediatr 1967;71:114–115.

10 Krams B, Echenne B, Leydet J, Rivier F, Roubertie A: Benign paroxysmal vertigo of childhood: long-term outcome. Cephalalgia 2010.

11 Cuvellier JC, Lepine A: Childhood periodic syndromes. Pediatr Neurol 2010;42: 1–11.

12 Lindskog U, Odkvist L, Noaksson L, Wallquist J: Benign paroxysmal vertigo in childhood: a long-term follow-up. Headache 1999;39:33–37.

13 Al-Twaijri WA, Shevell MI: Pediatric migraine equivalents: occurrence and clinical features in practice. Pediatr Neurol 2002;26:365–368.

14 Drigo P, Carli G, Laverda AM: Benign paroxysmal vertigo of childhood. Brain Dev 2001;23:38–41.
15 Lanzi G, Balottin U, Fazzi E, Tagliasacchi M, Manfrin M, Mira E: Benign paroxysmal vertigo of childhood: a long-term follow-up. Cephalalgia 1994;14:458–460.
16 Brantberg K, Trees N, Baloh RW: Migraine-associated vertigo. Acta Otolaryngol 2005;125:276–279.
17 Neuhauser HK, von Brevern M, Radtke A, Lezius F, Feldmann M, Ziese T, Lempert T: Epidemiology of vestibular vertigo: a neurotologic survey of the general population. Neurology 2005;65: 898–904.
18 Kayan A, Hood JD: Neuro-otological manifestations of migraine. Brain 1984; 107:1123–1142.
19 Lee H, Jen JC, Wang H, Chen Z, Mamsa H, Sabatti C, Baloh RW, Nelson SF: A genome-wide linkage scan of familial benign recurrent vertigo: linkage to 22q12 with evidence of heterogeneity. Hum Mol Genet 2006;15:251–258.
20 Migliaccio AA, Halmagyi GM, McGarvie LA, Cremer PD: Cerebellar ataxia with bilateral vestibulopathy: description of a syndrome and its characteristic clinical sign. Brain 2004;127:280–293.
21 Jen J, Baloh RH, Ishiyama A, Baloh RW: Dejerine-Sottas syndrome and vestibular loss due to a point mutation in the PMP22 gene. J Neurol Sci 2005;237:21–24.
22 Zingler VC, Cnyrim C, Jahn K, Weintz E, Fernbacher J, Frenzel C, Brandt T, Strupp M: Causative factors and epidemiology of bilateral vestibulopathy in 255 patients. Ann Neurol 2007;61:524–532.
23 Baloh RW, Jacobson K, Fife T: Familial vestibulopathy: a new dominantly inherited syndrome. Neurology 1994;44:20–25.
24 Brantberg K: Familial early-onset progressive vestibulopathy without hearing impairment. Acta Otolaryngol 2003;123: 713–717.
25 Verhagen WI, Huygen PL, Horstink MW: Familial congenital vestibular areflexia. J Neurol Neurosurg Psychiatry 1987;50: 933–935.
26 Jen JC, Wang H, Lee H, Sabatti C, Trent R, Hannigan I, Brantberg K, Halmagyi GM, Nelson SF, Baloh RW: Suggestive linkage to chromosome 6q in families with bilateral vestibulopathy. Neurology 2004;63:2376–2379.
27 Committee on Hearing and Equilibrium guidelines for the diagnosis and evaluation of therapy in Meniere's disease. Otolaryngol Head Neck Surg 1995;113: 181–185.
28 Bernstein JM: Occurrence of episodic vertigo and hearing loss in families. Ann Otol Rhinol Laryngol 1965;74:1011–1021.
29 Birgerson L, Gustavson KH, Stahle J: Familial Meniere's disease: a genetic investigation. Am J Otol 1987;8:323–326.
30 Frykholm C, Larsen HC, Dahl N, Klar J, Rask-Andersen H, Friberg U: Familial Meniere's disease in five generations. Otol Neurotol 2006;27:681–686.
31 Klockars T, Kentala E: Inheritance of Meniere's disease in the Finnish population. Arch Otolaryngol Head Neck Surg 2007;133:73–77.
32 Morrison AW: Anticipation in Meniere's disease. J Laryngol Otol 1995;109:499–502.
33 Morrison AW, Johnson KJ: Genetics (molecular biology) and Meniere's disease. Otolaryngol Clin North Am 2002; 35:497–516.
34 Oliveira CA, Ferrari I, Messias CI: Occurrence of familial Meniere's syndrome and migraine in Brasilia. Ann Otol Rhinol Laryngol 2002;111:229–236.
35 Brown M: Ménière's syndrome. Arch Neurol Psychiatry 1941;46:561–565.
36 Baloh R, Andrews J: Migraine and Ménière's disease; in Harris J (ed): Ménière's Disease. The Hague, Kugler Publications, 1999, pp 281–289.
37 Radtke A, Lempert T, Gresty MA, Brookes GB, Bronstein AM, Neuhauser H: Migraine and Meniere's disease: is there a link? Neurology 2002;59:1700–1704.
38 Robertson NG, Lu L, Heller S, Merchant SN, Eavey RD, McKenna M, Nadol JB Jr, Miyamoto RT, Linthicum FH Jr, Lubianca Neto JF, Hudspeth AJ, Seidman CE, Morton CC, Seidman JG: Mutations in a novel cochlear gene cause DFNA9, a human nonsyndromic deafness with vestibular dysfunction. Nat Genet 1998; 20:299–303.
39 Tamagawa Y, Ishikawa K, Ishikawa K, Ishida T, Kitamura K, Makino S, Tsuru T, Ichimura K: Phenotype of DFNA11: a nonsyndromic hearing loss caused by a myosin VIIA mutation. Laryngoscope 2002;112:292–297.
40 Fransen E, Verstreken M, Verhagen WI, Wuyts FL, Huygen PL, D'Haese P, Robertson NG, Morton CC, McGuirt WT, Smith RJ, Declau F, Van de Heyning PH, Van Camp G: High prevalence of symptoms of Meniere's disease in three families with a mutation in the COCH gene. Hum Mol Genet 1999;8:1425–1429.
41 Usami S, Takahashi K, Yuge I, Ohtsuka A, Namba A, Abe S, Fransen E, Patthy L, Otting G, Van Camp G: Mutations in the COCH gene are a frequent cause of autosomal dominant progressive cochleo-vestibular dysfunction, but not of Meniere's disease. Eur J Hum Genet 2003;11:744–748.
42 Sanchez E, Lopez-Escamez JA, Lopez-Nevot MA, Lopez-Nevot A, Cortes R, Martin J: Absence of COCH mutations in patients with Meniere disease. Eur J Hum Genet 2004;12:75–78.
43 Klar J, Frykholm C, Friberg U, Dahl N: A Meniere's disease gene linked to chromosome 12p12.3. Am J Med Genet B Neuropsychiatr Genet 2006;141:463–467.
44 Gabrikova D, Frykholm C, Friberg U, Lahsaee S, Entesarian M, Dahl N, Klar J: Familiar Meniere's disease restricted to 1.48 Mb on chromosome 12p12.3 by allelic and haplotype association. J Hum Genet 2010 Oct 7 [Epub ahead of print].

Joanna C. Jen
Department of Neurology, UCLA School of Medicine
710 Westwood Plaza
Los Angeles, CA 90095-1769 (USA)
Tel. +1 310 825 3731, Fax +1 310 206 1513, E-Mail jjen@ucla.edu

Alford RL, Sutton VR (eds): Medical Genetics in the Clinical Practice of ORL.
Adv Otorhinolaryngol. Basel, Karger, 2011, vol 70, pp 135–140

Genetics of Otitis Media

J. Christopher Post

Pediatric Otolaryngology, and Center for Genomic Sciences, Allegheny General Hospital, Pittsburgh, Pa., USA

Abstract

There is a growing body of evidence, both from animal and human studies, that host genetic factors can influence the risk of developing otitis media (OM). The role of genetics in OM has been elucidated through studies with monozygotic and dizygotic twins, analyses linking genetic polymorphisms to OM susceptibility, and genome scans. Several twin studies have shown a strong genetic component to middle ear effusion risk, with the estimate of the role of heredity for the proportion of time with middle ear effusions being around 0.7. Genetic polymorphisms in plasminogen activator inhibitor-1, interleukin-6, tumor necrosis factor-α, human leukocyte antigen, and mannose-binding lectin have been variously linked with OM and upper respiratory infection susceptibility. Several genome linkage studies have identified chromosomal regions associated with chronic OM, including 3p, 10q, 10q22.3, 17q12 and 19q. A number of candidate genes are associated with these sites. Given the current state of understanding of the role of genetics in OM, a family history of OM should be ascertained for all patients. Children with a strong family history of OM should be considered as candidates for a more aggressive early treatment of OM, particularly if other risk factors are present. These children may be earlier candidates for the placement of tympanostomy tubes and/or adenoidectomy. Existing data do not support routine genetic testing to determine a child's susceptibility to OM; however, given the advances in whole genome sequencing, such testing may someday play a role in the management of the OM patient.

While most children are exposed to viral rhinosinusitis, the likelihood of developing acute otitis media (OM) depends on demographic, environmental, and genetic factors [1]. Many of these factors likewise influence the risk for persistent OM with effusion, including frequent acute OM and upper respiratory infections, parental smoking, exposure to daycare centers, allergy history, number of siblings, and poor educational status in parents. Genetics and family history may be especially important factors for determining risk for OM and aggressiveness with which OM should be treated.

Animal models have been used to help identify genetic mechanisms of increased OM susceptibility [2]. For example, genetic changes affecting both ear anatomy [3] and immune defense mechanisms [4] have been related to increased OM risk in mice. A wide range of human studies have likewise supported an important role of genetics in OM susceptibility.

Genetics of Otitis Media

Understanding genetic factors in OM is important because of the high prevalence of OM and consequences of recurrent ear infections.

Numerous genetic studies have been conducted over the last several decades to identify inherited risk factors for OM. Genetically controlled differences in anatomy (e.g. variations in the structure of the Eustachian tube and the rate of development of the nasopharynx) and immunologic factors (e.g. cytokines and mucins) likely contribute to the heritable nature of recurrent OM [5]. Furthermore, a variety of candidates genes linked to recurrent OM susceptibility have been identified (table 1) [6]. The role of genetics in OM has been elucidated through twin studies, analyses linking polymorphisms to OM susceptibility, and genome scans. Current data for each type of analysis are described below.

Twin Studies
Twins studies can be particularly helpful in determining the role of genetics, as monozygotic twins share the same DNA sequence, while only about 50% is shared by dizygotic twins. A landmark longitudinal study by Casselbrandt et al. [7] followed twins and triplets ≤2 months old for up to 2 years. This study showed a strong genetic component to the amount of time children experienced middle ear effusions, as well as episodes of effusion and acute OM. Contribution from inheritance was estimated in this study as 0.73 overall, with estimates of 0.64 for males and 0.79 for females ($p < 0.001$ for each).

A more recent, 5-year, prospective study by this same group followed babies from sets of twins and triplets with monthly otoscopy and tympanometry examinations to calculate the time with middle ear effusions [8]. Comparisons were made between time with effusions for monozygotic and dizygotic sets. The estimate of the role of heredity for the proportion of time with middle ear effusions for this 5-year period was 0.72 ($p < 0.001$). Correlation of the cumulative proportion of time with middle ear effusions was higher in monozygotic sets (0.65–0.81) compared with dizygotic sets (0.28–0.40). These differences showed a trend during the first year ($p = 0.06$), with significance

Table 1. Candidate genes linked to OM susceptibility (based on Casselbrandt 2005)

Cytokine genes (TNF-α, and IFN-γ)
G immunoglobulin receptor gene (Fc receptors)
Surfactant protein genes (e.g. pulmonary-surfactant associated protein gene)
Mucin gene upregulation (e.g. mucin 2)
Cathepsin protease gene upregulation (e.g. cathepsin B)

during the remaining 4 years ($p < 0.001$). For noncumulative correlations analyzed each year independently, the correlation was significantly higher during the first 3 years in monozygotic sets (0.65–0.77) compared with dizygotic sets (0.31–0.39). The strength of this correlation decreased during years 4 and 5. Noncumulative correlations for monozygotic and dizygotic sets, respectively, were 0.31 and 0.05 in year 4 and –0.04 and –0.14 during year 5; neither of these differences was statistically significant. These data support a strong genetic component to middle ear effusion risk during the first 3 years of life, which becomes less pronounced after age 3.

Another longitudinal study using a Norwegian database likewise correlated shared genetics with increased risk for recurrent OM in a sample of 4,247 twin pairs [9]. Tetrachoric correlation for recurrent OM is shown in figure 1. In this study, genetic effects estimated about 70% of the OM risk, 72% in males and 61% in females. Similarly, a longitudinal study of same-sex twins born in England or Wales related high scores for symptoms of middle ear disease with genetics [10]. At age 2, proband concordance was 95% among monozygotic twins and 63% in dyzygotic twins. Concordance for high middle ear disease symptoms in monozygotic and dizygotic twins, respectively, were 91% and 67% at age 3 and 85% and 68% at age 4. Acute infections items showed an overall lower heritability than chronic symptoms.

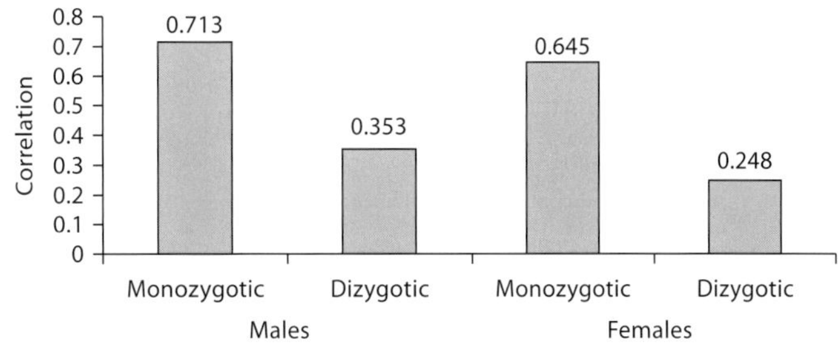

Fig. 1. Tetrachoric correlation of recurrent OM before age 7 (Based on Kvestad et al. [9]). Correlation values can vary from –1 (perfect negative correlation) to 0 (no correlation) to +1 (perfect positive correlation). For both male and female twin pairs, positive correlation for recurrent OM was greater (with values closer to 1) for monozygotic twins.

Polymorphisms and OM Susceptibility

Plasminogen Activator Inhibitor-1

In addition to its important role in fibrinolysis, plasminogen activator inhibitor-1 (PAI-1) is an important inhibitor of tissue repair [11]. The PAI-1 gene is located at 7q21.3-q22. The PAI-1 4G/5G promoter polymorphism results in the slightly less active 5G allele. Because the 4G allele produces more PAI-1, tissue repair is reduced in those with this genotype. Genotyping a sample of Dutch children linked the PAI-1 (4G) genotype with increased risk for more frequent episodes of acute OM compared with children who were homozygous for the 5G allele [12].

Cytokine Genes

Proinflammatory cytokine polymorphisms for interleukin (IL)-6^{-174} and tumor necrosis factor-α $(TNFα)^{-308}$ have been retrospectively linked with OM susceptibility and tympanostomy tube placement [13]. These same polymorphisms have also been linked to OM in a prospective study [14]. DNA cytokine genotypes were identified in 242 children followed for 1 year for the occurrence of upper respiratory tract infection and acute OM. Children with the IL-6^{-174} polymorphism were 24% more likely to have upper respiratory tract infections, while the $TNFα^{-308}$ polymorphism was not linked to upper respiratory infection risk. Having either IL-6^{-174} or $TNFα^{-308}$ polymorphism, however, doubled the risk of being susceptible to OM (OR 2.1, 95% CI 1.1–3.8). Furthermore, children with the $TNFα^{-308}$ polymorphism had a 42% greater risk of developing acute OM after an upper respiratory infection, while this risk was not increased among children with the IL-6^{-174} polymorphism.

The significance of various cytokine polymorphisms and risk for developing OM after an upper respiratory infection was analyzed in a 4-year study of 205 children between ages 1 and 5 years and their older siblings who were <10 years old [15]. Odds ratios for OM occurring with upper respiratory infection for several significant demographic and phenotypic characteristics are shown in figure 2. Significant predictors of new episodes of OM occurring during upper respiratory infections were: younger age; a history of OM, a daily environment other than being home with mother; high production of IL-10 and TNFα phenotypes; and low production IL-6 phenotype.

Human Leukocyte Antigens

Human leukocyte antigens (HLA) polymorphism may also be linked to OM risk. Two older studies by the same research group showed differences in hereditary influence from HLA antigens on recurrent acute and chronic secretory OM [16, 17]. While the prevalence of HLA-A2 was higher in children with recurrent acute OM compared with controls (80 vs. 56%) and HLA-A3 was lower (11

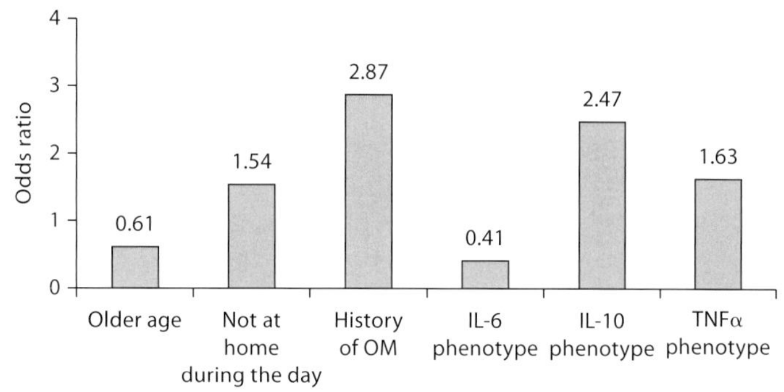

Fig. 2. Significant predictors of OM occurring with upper respiratory infections (Based on Alper et al. [15]). All factors shown were statistically significant ($p \leq 0.05$). Odds ratio <1 denotes reduced risk; odds ratio >1 signifies increased risk for developing OM when the child experienced an upper respiratory infection with rhinovirus.

vs. 28%) [16], the proportions of HLA-A2 and HLA-A3 in children with chronic secretory OM (52 and 28%, respectively) were similar to those for controls [17].

Mannose-Binding Lectin

Mannose-binding lectin (MBL) is an important immune factor that activates the complement system. MBL polymorphisms have generally been inconsistently linked to upper respiratory infection susceptibility in children [18]. Recently, MBL2 polymorphisms have been linked to susceptibility for respiratory tract infections in young men [19] and a new study evaluating MBL2 gene polymorphisms identified a significantly higher frequency of the promoter LXP haplotype and B allele in children with recurrent respiratory infections compared with controls [20]. The LXP haplotype has been linked to low MBL levels [21] and indeed children with recurrent respiratory infections in the current study also had significantly lower MBL levels [20]. The role of MBL polymorphisms in otitis media has not been specifically studied.

Genome Scan in Children Needing Tympanostomy Tube Insertion

Daly et al. [22] evaluated 588 individuals who had undergone tympanostomy tube insertion for chronic/recurrent OM with DNA analysis. Three distinct chromosomal regions were identified as important influences (table 2). Both nonparametric and parametric analyses supported linkages between regions on chromosomes 10q and 19q with chronic/recurrent OM, with conditional analyses revealing an interactive site between these two regions and chromosome 3p. These data suggest that individuals might inherit anatomical or immunological factors that increase their susceptibility to the development of clinical OM when exposed to microbes [22].

Recently, Casselbrandt et al. [23] conducted a genome linkage scan of full siblings with a history of tympanostomy tube insertion due to OM and their family members. A total of 403 Caucasian families with 1,431 individuals were genotyped. Their study identified significant linkages at 10q22.3 and 17q12. Possible candidate genes at these sites are pulmonary-surfactant associated protein gene SFTPA2 in the 10q22.3 region and adaptor-related protein complex 2, beta 1 subunit (AP2B1) and chemokine ligand 5 (CCL5; also called RANTES) in the 17q12 region. AP2B1 encodes a protein in coated vesicles and plays a role in CD8 killer cell downregulation that has been implicated in recurrent OM [24]. Cytokines are involved in immunoregulatory and inflammatory processes. CCL5 has also been implicated in OM with effusion [25].

Table 2. OM susceptibility loci (based on Daly et al. [22])

Chromosome	Affected region	Number of genes encoded on affected region	Gene region function
10q	D10S212	25	Killer cell immunoglobulin-like receptors that regulate cytotoxic activity of natural killer and some T cells Immunoglobulin-like transcripts that prevent activation of immune cells
19q	D19S254	28	ADAM8 allergen-induced asthma gene is in this region
3p	between D3S4545 and D3S1259	2	Inflammatory mediators histamine receptor H1 and IL-1 receptor-activated kinase 2

Applying Genetics to Clinical Practice

A family history of OM should be carefully ascertained for all children. Patients with a strong family history of OM may require more aggressive early treatment of OM, particularly if other risk factors, such as frequent exposure to infections (e.g. daycare exposure) or parental smoking, are also present. Parents with a history of recurrent OM should be counseled to minimize exposure to other risk factors in their children, including respiratory inhalants and others with acute respiratory infections. In addition, children with OM who have a strong family history may be earlier candidates for tympanostomy tubes and adenoidectomy. While adenoidectomy is typically reserved for more recalcitrant infections, adenoidectomy may be considered earlier in the course of OM treatment in children with a strong genetic history, e.g. a family history of recurrent OM. Furthermore, genetically high-risk children may constitute an appropriate group for routine use of OM vaccines [26].

Role of Genetic Testing

The existing data do not support a role for genetic testing in the management of OM; however, advances in technology and a richer understanding of the genetics of OM may some day enable the routine use of genetic testing to identify risk. Further investigations into the genetics of OM will certainly enhance the understanding of the underlying pathophysiology of the disease, and suggest additional management strategies.

References

1 Gultekin E, Develioğlu ON, Yener M, Ozdemir I, Külekci M: Prevalence and risk factors for persistent otitis media with effusion in primary school children in Istanbul, Turkey. Auris Nasus Larynx. In press.

2 Trune DR, Zheng QY: Mouse models for human otitis media. Brain Res 2009; 1277:90–103.

3 Depreux FF, Darrow K, Conner DA, et al: Eya4-deficient mice are a model for heritable otitis media. J Clin Invest 2008; 118:471–474.

4 Hernandez M, Leichtle A, Pak K, et al: Myeloid differentiation primary response gene 88 is required for the resolution of otitis media. J Infect Dis 2008; 198:1862–1869.

5 Casselbrandt ML, Mandel EM: The genetics of otitis media. Curr Allergy Asthma Rep 2001;1:353–357.
6 Casselbrandt ML, Mandel EM: Genetic susceptibility to otitis media. Curr Opin Allergy Clin Immunol 2005;5:1–4.
7 Casselbrandt ML, Mandel EM, Fall PA, et al: The heritability of otitis media: a twin and triplet study. JAMA 1999;282: 2125–2130.
8 Casselbrandt ML, Mandel EM, Rockette HE, et al: The genetic component of middle ear disease in the first 5 years of life. Arch Otolaryngol Head Neck Surg 2004;130:273–278.
9 Kvestad E, Kværner KJ, Røysamb E, et al: Otitis media: genetic factors and sex differences. Twin Res 2004;7:239–244.
10 Rovers M, Haggard M, Gannon M, Koeppen-Schomerus G, Plomin R: Heritability of symptom domains in otitis media: a longitudinal study of 1,373 twin pairs. Am J Epidemiol 2002;155: 958–964.
11 Lijnen HR: Pleiotropic functions of plasminogen activator inhibitor-1. J Thromb Haemost 2005;3:35–45.
12 Emonts M, Wiertsma SP, Veenhoven RH, et al: The 4G/4G plasminogen activator inhibitor-1 genotype is associated with frequent recurrence of acute otitis media. Pediatrics 2007;120:e317–e323.
13 Patel JA, Nair S, Revai K, et al: Association of proinflammatory cytokine gene polymorphisms with susceptibility to otitis media. Pediatrics 2006;118:2273–2279.
14 Revai K, Patel JA, Grady JJ, et al: Association between cytokine gene polymorphisms and risk for upper respiratory tract infection and acute otitis media. Clin Infect Dis 2009;49:257–261.
15 Alper CM, Winther B, Hendley JO, Doyle WJ: Cytokine polymorphisms predict the frequency of otitis media as a complication of rhinovirus and RSV infections in children. Eur Arch Otorhinolaryngol 2009;266:199–205.
16 Kalm O, Johnson U, Prellner K, Ninn K: HLA frequency in patients with recurrent acute otitis media. Arch Otolaryngol Head Neck Surg 1991;117:1296–1299.
17 Kalm O, Johnson U, Prellner K: HLA frequency in patients with chronic secretory otitis media. Int J Pediatr Otorhinolaryngol 1994;30:151–157.
18 Ruskamp JM, Hoekstra MO, Rovers MM, Schilder AG, Sanders EA: Mannose-binding lectin and upper respiratory tract infections in children and adolescents: a review. Arch Otolaryngol Head Neck Surg 2006;132:482–486.
19 Rantala A, Lajunen T, Juvonen R, et al: Mannose-binding lectin concentrations, MBL2 polymorphisms, and susceptibility to respiratory tract infections in young men. J Infect Dis 2008;198:1247–1253.
20 Chen J, Xu Z, Ou X, et al: Mannose-binding lectin polymorphisms and recurrent respiratory tract infection in Chinese children. Eur J Pediatr 2009; 168:1305–1313.
21 Madsen HO, Garred P, Thiel S, et al: Interplay between promoter and structural gene variants control basal serum level of mannan-binding protein. J Immunol 1995;155:3013–3020.
22 Daly KA, Brown WM, Segade F, et al: Chronic and recurrent otitis media: a genome scan for susceptibility loci. Am J Hum Genet 2004;75:988–997.
23 Casselbrandt ML, Mandel EM, Jung J, et al: Otitis media: a genome-wide linkage scan with evidence of susceptibility loci within the 17q12 and 10q22.3 regions. BMC Med Genetics 2009;10:85.
24 Avanzini AM, Castellazzi AM, Marconi M, et al: Children with recurrent otitis show defective IFN gamma-producing cells in adenoids. Pediatr Allergy Immunol 2008;19:523–526.
25 Schousboe LP, Rasumussen LM, Ovesen T: RANTES in otitis media with effusion: presence, role and correlation with cytokines and microbiology. APMIS 2001;109:441–446.
26 O'Brien MA, Prosser LA, Paradise JL, et al: New vaccines against otitis media: projected benefits and cost-effectiveness. Pediatrics 2009;123:1452–1463.

J. Christopher Post, MD
Allegheny General Hospital
320 East North Avenue
Pittsburgh, PA 15212 (USA)
Tel. +1 412 359 5163, Fax +1 412 359 6995, E-Mail cpost@wpahs.org

Alford RL, Sutton VR (eds): Medical Genetics in the Clinical Practice of ORL.
Adv Otorhinolaryngol. Basel, Karger, 2011, vol 70, pp 141–151

Gene Therapy for Head and Neck Cancer

Waleed M. Abuzeid[a] · Daqing Li[b] · Bert W. O'Malley Jr.[b]

[a]Department of Otolaryngology, Head & Neck Surgery, University of Michigan, Ann Arbor, Mich., and [b]Department of Otorhinolaryngology, Head & Neck Surgery, University of Pennsylvania School of Medicine, Philadelphia, Pa., USA

Abstract

The mortality associated with head and neck cancer has remained largely unchanged for the past several decades despite advancements in surgery, radiotherapy and chemotherapy. Gene therapy is a novel treatment approach that may potentially advance the treatment of genetic diseases, which include malignancies such as head and neck cancer. Multiple vector systems have been developed that facilitate the introduction of therapeutic genetic material into cells. These include DNA-based vectors, viral vectors and, most recently, vectors that induce RNA interference. Gene therapy strategies can be classified in 3 groups: (1) cytoreductive therapy aimed at directly inducing cell death, (2) corrective therapy intended to repair genetic defects underlying malignancy, and (3) immune modulation to promote a robust immune response against cancer cells. Translational research has been conducted in each of these areas, culminating in clinical trials and the implementation of gene therapy as a viable therapeutic modality for head and neck cancers.

Gene therapy is the treatment of disease through the introduction of genetic material into cells in order to treat or prevent disease. Initial gene therapy trials involved the introduction of a wild-type gene into somatic cells in order to correct disease caused by a single, identifiable gene defect. For example, severe combined immunodeficiency has been effectively treated through the introduction of a functioning adenine deaminase gene into the bone marrow of affected children [1].

In recent years, there has been an increasing realization that cancer is also a genetic disease. This is based on the observation that epigenetic and genetic mutations in somatic cells, the vast majority of which are spontaneous rather than inherited, initiate cancer [2]. Cancer cells share certain key features: insensitivity to anti-growth signals, autonomous pro-growth signals, enhancement of angiogenesis, evasion of apoptosis, locoregional invasion and metastasis, and immortality [2]. These features are, essentially, the targets for novel gene therapy treatments.

Head and neck cancer represents an ideal target for gene therapy. Globally, over 500,000 cases are diagnosed per year [3]. Head and neck cancer is normally treated with surgery or radiotherapy, alone or in combination, and, in addition, adjuvant or concurrent chemotherapy is often added for more advanced disease. Despite developments in these standard treatments, the overall 5-year survival rate for newly diagnosed head and neck cancer has remained at 50–60% over the past three decades [4]. At diagnosis, head and neck cancer is usually limited to the primary site or cervical lymph nodes, both of which often lie in or close to skin or mucosal surfaces, ideally positioned for intratumoral injection of gene therapy vectors [3].

Gene therapy treatments can be grouped into: (1) cytoreductive therapy to directly induce cancer cell death, (2) corrective therapy to correct an underlying cancer-inducing genetic defect, or (3) immune modulation to facilitate the host response to cancer cells. Before detailing these approaches, a discussion about the vectors used to deliver therapeutic genes is warranted.

Vectors

DNA-Based Vectors

Early experiments in gene therapy utilized DNA to insert or 'transfect' genes into the chromosomes of target cells. The desired genes are packaged into circular molecules of DNA-termed plasmids which are capable of replication independent of chromosomal DNA, allowing them to sustain gene expression for longer periods of time than is possible with linear DNA. Plasmids incorporate modifiable promoter and enhancer sequences that initiate and regulate the rate of gene transcription, respectively.

Various methods exist for transferring plasmids into target cells. In vitro techniques include microinjection of plasmids directly into cell nuclei [5]. In vivo plasmid transfer can, in its simplest form, be accomplished through direct injection of target tissues. Direct plasmid injection has been successfully used in clinical trials for malignant melanoma [6]. Injecting plasmids into tissues using high velocity air or fluids also enhances transfection, so-called bio-ballistics [7]. Similarly, the 'gene gun' accelerates plasmid-coated gold particles into target tissues [8]. The relatively superficial location of most head and neck cancers makes them amenable to electroporation through surface electrode placement. Electroporation utilizes electric current to transiently increase the permeability of the cell membrane. The safety and efficacy of electroporation for gene transfer was recently demonstrated in a clinical trial involving patients with metastatic malignant melanoma [9]. Plasmids can be incorporated into a liposomal carrier vehicle that protects the enclosed DNA from degradation and can be designed with DNA-tropic characteristics. This method has been used to successfully induce significant tumor kill through transfection of the immunomodulatory IL-2 gene or cytotoxic E1A gene into murine head and neck squamous cell carcinoma (HNSCC) models and in humans [10–12].

The inherent advantages of plasmid-gene therapy include the modifiable duration of gene expression from several hours to many months [13, 14]. Permanent alteration to the host genome is avoided. Clinical scenarios amenable to short-term gene expression are ideally treated with plasmid therapy. Similarly, if a particular disease process necessitates periods of short-term gene expression, repeat injection of plasmids is feasible as there is no significant systemic inflammatory response. An ongoing problem with plasmid-based vectors is traditionally low transfection efficiency.

Viral Vectors

Viruses have evolved to infect host cells and to commandeer their biosynthetic mechanisms for subsequent replication, packaging and release. An ideal viral vector is capable of infecting cancer cells and inducing sustainable gene expression while concurrently limiting damage to normal cells. Achieving this goal involves modifying the viral genome to include the therapeutic gene and the native genes necessary for attachment, penetration and transgene expression, but lacking the genes involved in replication, which are often the same genes that cause pathogenicity [3]. These replication-deficient viruses cannot propagate but retain the ability to induce transgene expression. Viral tropism can also be modified by augmenting

Table 1. Viral vectors for gene therapy

	Adenovirus	Retrovirus	Lentivirus	Adeno-associated virus	Herpesvirus
Infection specificity	broad	dividing cells only	broad	dividing and non-dividing cells	dividing cells only
Transgene integration site	episomal	nonspecific chromosomal	nonspecific chromosomal	specific chromosomal	episomal
Duration of transgene expression	transient	stable	stable	stable	transient
Maximal gene carrying capacity	large (~36 kb) with 'gutless' vectors	intermediate (~10 kb)	intermediate (~10 kb)	small (~5 kb)	large (~36 kb)
Achievable viral titers	high	low	low	low	low
Risks	innate immune response (minimal with newer vectors)	insertional mutagenesis	insertional mutagenesis	contamination of clinical stock with helper virus; adaptive immune response	innate and adaptive immune response

or replacing viral surface receptors involved in cell binding and internalization with ligands that recognize receptors up-regulated in cancer such as the coxsackie and adenovirus receptor [15]. Specificity can also be enhanced through the use of cancer specific promoters such as telomerase promoter. Telomerase is over-expressed in many HNSCC cells, effectively limiting transgene expression to malignant cells [16, 17]. Table 1 summarizes the key characteristics of different viral vectors which are discussed in detail below.

Retroviruses

Retrovirus vectors irreversibly integrate the therapeutic gene into the host genome producing permanent gene expression. This characteristic underlies retrovirus-induced insertional oncogenesis where nearby proto-oncogenes are activated through genomic integration. Indeed, several children receiving curative gene therapy for SCID developed T cell leukemia many years later [18]. Insertional oncogenesis can potentially be prevented through the use of insulator genes to isolate the transgene from the cellular genome. Alternatively, suicide genes can be integrated along with the therapeutic gene to terminate overproliferating cells [19]. Retroviruses will only integrate into actively dividing cells limiting their use in cancers where a proportion of cells are often latent. This limitation can be overcome through the use of retrovirus-related lentivirus vectors which can permanently integrate genes into nondividing cells [2].

Retroviruses have been used to treat thyroid cancer in a murine model through immunomodulation and suicide gene approaches [20]. There have been no clinical trials to date treating HNSCC with retroviruses but clinical trials in other areas suggest that these viruses are, generally, safe [21–23].

Adenoviruses

Adenoviruses remain episomal and, unlike retroviral vectors, do not integrate their genes into the host cell chromosome reducing the risk of insertional oncogenesis. Additionally, adenovirus vectors can infect both dividing cells and nondividing cells. The transgene expression efficiency is significantly higher than is achievable with plasmids [24, 25]. First-generation adenovirus vectors included deletions to render them replication deficient but contained enough of their native genome to render them highly immunogenic, which carries the risk of immune mediated toxicity and even patient death [26, 27]. Later generation adenoviruses included deletions of the E1A, E2A, E3 and E4 viral genes, markedly reducing immunogenicity while maintaining infection efficiency [26, 28]. The newest 'gutless' adenovirus vectors contain a bare minimum of viral genes rendering them even less inflammatory and thus significantly reducing the viral associated toxicities [3].

Over 200 clinical trials in the US alone have utilized adenovirus vectors with minimal toxicity demonstrated in all but a few cases. This suggests that these vectors, particularly later generation variants, are safe for human use [26].

Other Viral Vectors

Replication-deficient adeno-associated viruses (AAV) can permanently integrate the transgene into the host genome of dividing and nondividing cells. Transgene insertion occurs at predictable sites reducing the risk of insertional oncogenesis [29]. However, AAV vectors have an extremely limited gene carrying capacity and require a cytotoxic helper virus to produce clinically effective quantities of vector [3]. The need for and use of helper virus raises the risk of viral contamination to the human clinical grade treatment stock, which limits the excitement and clinical applicability of this vector for use in humans.

Replication-competent herpes simplex virus (HSV) has modified virulence genes rendering it dependent upon the cell machinery of actively dividing cells for replication, conferring safety and some degree of cancer selectivity. HSV is inherently cytotoxic as the replicative life cycle of the virus destroys the host cell [30]. Second-generation HSV vectors contain multiple mutations intended to overcome dose-limiting toxicities. HSV vectors, in combination with cisplatin, have proven efficacy against HNSCC in murine models, achieving 100% cure in certain cell lines [31]. Phase I trials using replication-competent HSV harboring granulocyte-macrophage colony-stimulating factor (GM-CSF), intended to enhance the host cell immune response against the infected cell, have shown low toxicity and excellent antitumor efficacy [32].

RNA-Based Vectors

Researchers have previously noted that suppression of key oncogenes can induce tumor regression. Recently, the new technology of 'RNA interference' has emerged that can effectively 'silence' any gene [33] (fig. 1). The key effector in RNA interference is a short sequence of 21 nucleotides, so called small interfering RNA (siRNA), which binds to complementary mRNA sequences, triggering cleavage of the mRNA and failure of transcription. Sub-nanomolar concentrations of siRNA can suppress mRNA levels by over 90% [34]. However, siRNA is susceptible to 'off-target' effects in which unintended gene silencing occurs. Sequence homology between the siRNA and host genes of as little as seven base pairs is enough to induce an off-target effect. However, this potential drawback has not been observed in human clinical trials of RNA interference which demonstrate excellent tolerability [35].

The delivery of siRNA to target tissues continues to present a challenge. Initial investigations involved intravenous administration. However, naked siRNA has a half-life of only 0.03 hours resulting in a transient therapeutic effect. This can be enhanced

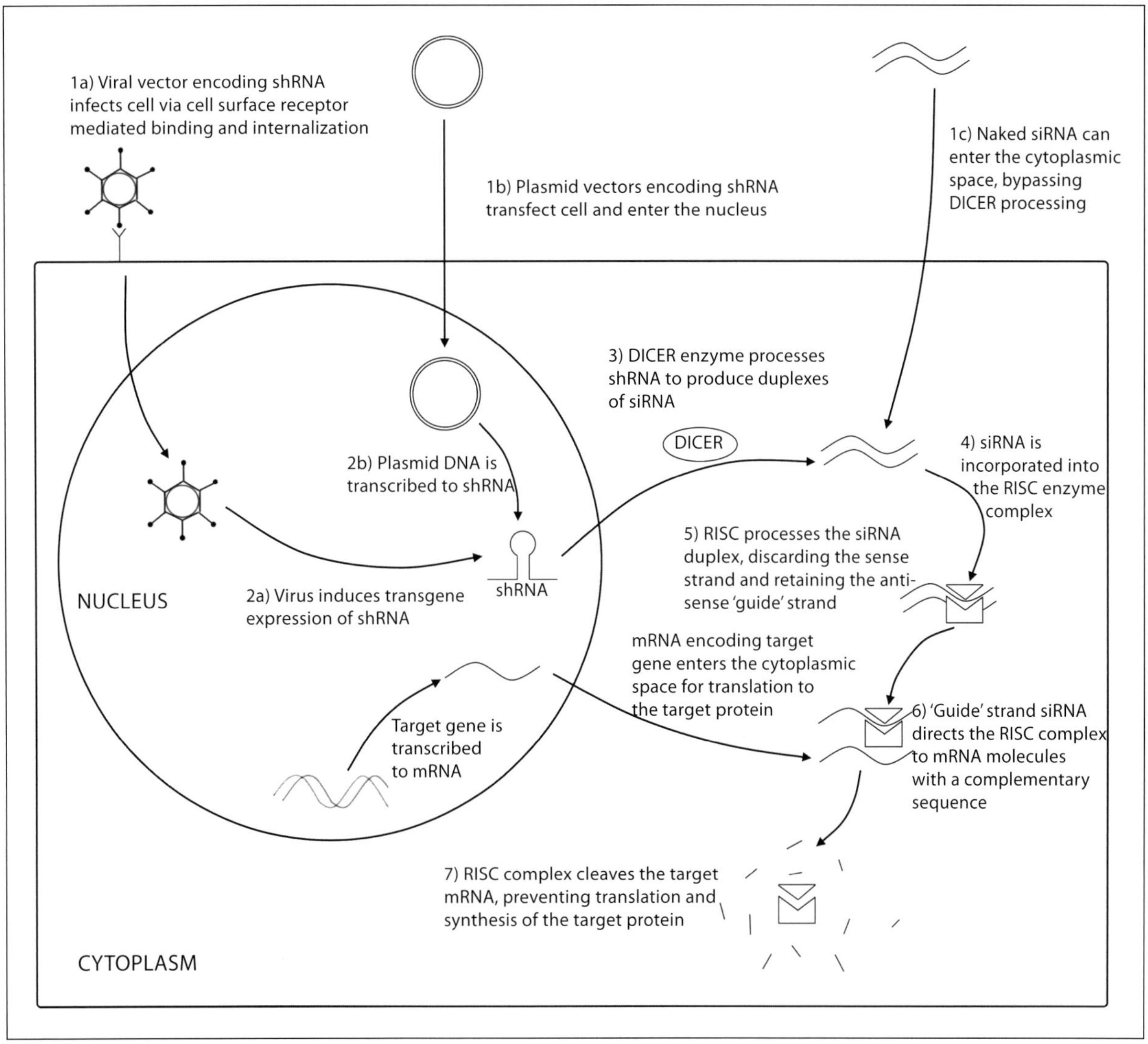

Fig. 1. Mechanisms of RNA interference. A viral (1a, 2a) or plasmid (1b, 2b) vector can be used to introduce shRNA into the cell which undergoes further processing by Dicer (3) to yield siRNA. Alternatively, naked siRNA (1c) can bypass Dicer processing entirely. Cytoplasmic siRNA is incorporated into the RISC complex (4) and further processed to yield an anti-sense 'guide' strand (5). This permits the activated RISC complex to 'home in' to mRNA molecules with a sequence complementary to the 'guide' strand (6). The target mRNA is then cleaved preventing translation to the target protein (7). In this way, the target gene is effectively 'silenced'.

to 6.5 h by conjugating the siRNA to lipid [36]. This translates to a therapeutic effect lasting from hours to a few days – a duration not conducive to cancer treatment. Gene silencing can be markedly prolonged by using liposomes to deliver siRNA [37]. Nanoparticles consisting of a cationic polymer to bind the siRNA and protect the sequence from degradation, a 'stealth' coating to overcome immune surveillance and a targeting ligand to 'home' the particle in on target tissues, have been designed and used to silence VEGF and effect tumor involution [38]. Hydrodynamic bio-ballistics remains the most popular method for introducing siRNA into tissues [39]. DNA plasmids have been used to deliver genes encoding special double-stranded RNA molecules – short-hairpin RNA (shRNA) – containing a sharp hairpin turn that facilitates intracellular processing into siRNA. These shRNA-encoding DNA plasmids can prolong the duration of gene silencing to several weeks, but can transfect only nondividing cells [35, 40]. This limitation has recently been overcome by using viral vectors, such as adenovirus, to incorporate and induce transgene expression of shRNA [35].

Gene Therapy Approaches

Cytoreductive Gene Therapy

One of the earliest approaches to inducing a direct cytotoxic effect was through suicide gene therapy. This concept involves the delivery of genes encoding specific enzymes into cancer cells. These enzymes then metabolize inactive pro-drugs to active, toxic metabolites creating a tumor-specific chemotherapeutic effect. The most common system involves transgene expression of thymidine kinase derived from the herpes simplex virus (HSV-Tk) in cancer cells followed by administration of the antiviral drug, ganciclovir, which is metabolized by HSV-Tk to a cytotoxic metabolite [41] (fig. 2). HSV-Tk delivery was initially accomplished with a retroviral vector but the inherently low infection efficiency prompted the use of replication-defective adenovirus vectors. Recent advances have resulted in the development of HNSCC-targeted adenoviral vectors harboring the HSV-Tk gene with a significant antitumor effect both in vitro and in animals [42]. The first Phase I clinical trial using HSV-Tk against head and neck malignancies was recently completed. Although the treatment was well tolerated, with fever being the main adverse reaction, patients only exhibited a mild-to-moderate tumor response [41]. The unimpressive clinical response is likely due to the use of direct antitumor injection. Dissemination of the virus throughout the tumor is compromised, particularly in large, bulky HNSCC primaries, and this will limit therapeutic efficacy.

Recent advancements have led to targeted suicide gene therapy vectors through exploitation of the inherent genetic differences between cancer and normal cells. This led to the development of conditionally replicating viruses which selectively infect and replicate in cells that have a specific genetic defect such as loss of p53 gene expression – a common event in head and neck cancers. Normal cells harboring active p53 are left untouched. ONYX-015, a conditionally replicating adenovirus, lacks the gene encoding the p53 binding gene, E1B-55kDa. The product of this gene binds to and inactivates cellular p53, a key step in initiation of viral replication. ONYX-015, therefore, demonstrates a bias for replication in p53-deficient cells [3, 43]. Nonetheless, ONYX-015 has not proven particularly effective as a monotherapy in phase II trials of recurrent head and neck cancer with response rates of only 15% [44, 45]. However, in human clinical trials combining ONYX-015 and cisplatin or 5-fluorouracil, a significant number of complete clinical responses were achieved whereas tumors treated with chemotherapy alone universally progressed [46]. These results were replicated in a randomized phase III clinical trial in China utilizing H101, a virus similar to ONYX-015, in which patients with locally advanced head and neck cancers who were treated with H101 and chemotherapy showed a significantly higher response rate than those treated with chemotherapy alone [47]. More recently designed conditionally replicating adenoviruses include OBP-401 where a human telomerase reverse transcriptase (hTERT) activated promoter drives the transcription of the viral E1 gene, activating viral replication and inducing cytolysis. Human TERT is the catalytic subunit of telomerase which is activated in over 90% of HNSCC. OBP-401 is, therefore, preferentially activated in cancer cells. In vivo, OBP-401 not only successfully

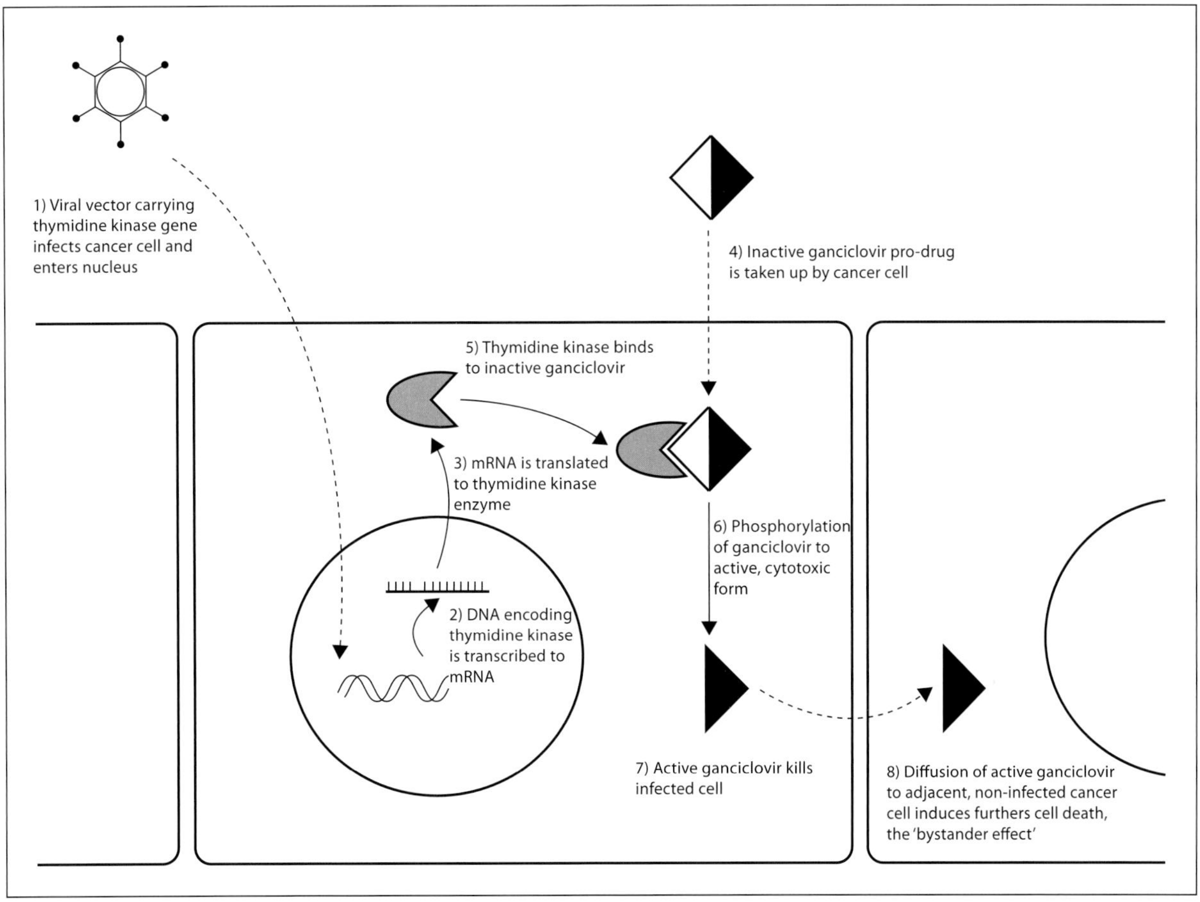

Fig. 2. Suicide gene therapy using thymidine kinase in combination with ganciclovir. The most common variant of this system uses a herpes simplex virus encoding the thymidine kinase gene that infects the target cancer cell (1). The gene is transcribed to mRNA (2) and translated to the active enzyme (3). Ganciclovir, a non-cytotoxic pro-drug, is concurrently administered and taken up by the target cancer cell (4). The thymidine kinase enzyme binds to (5) and phosphorylates ganciclovir to its cytotoxic form (6). This cytotoxic metabolite not only kills the infected target cancer cell (7), but can diffuse across cell membranes to adjacent, uninfected cells inducing further cell death - the so-called 'bystander effect' (8).

treated HNSCC at the primary site but also 'homed in' on cancer cells that had metastasized via lymphatics to lymph nodes, obliterating cancer cells at these locations and, by tagging the virus with a fluorescent marker, acting as a diagnostic modality to track cancer spread in real-time [48].

Other cytoreductive strategies are in development. The disruption of DNA repair mechanisms can sensitize HNSCC to cisplatin, permitting the use of lower, less toxic doses of this standard therapy while simultaneously enhancing tumor kill [49]. Targeting angiogenic mechanisms may hold promise as tumors cannot grow beyond 1–2 mm without recruiting a blood supply through angiogenesis [50, 51]. Vascular endothelial growth factor (VEGF) is overexpressed in many head and neck cancers and elevated pretreatment levels have been associated with tumor progression, poor treatment response and reduced survival [52]. The inhibition of VEGF using plasmid-delivered shRNA has been shown to significantly enhance laryngeal SCC cell death [53, 54]. Mechanisms that confer immortality to cancer cells can also be targeted. For example, Bcl-xl is a potent anti-apoptotic gene that is overexpressed in many cancers and knockdown of this gene dramatically increases the proportion of laryngeal cancer cells undergoing apoptosis [54]. Telomerase also contributed to cancer cell immortality through the maintenance of telomere length. Gene silencing of hTERT induces an approximate 80% reduction in HNSCC growth in vitro and in vivo [53]. Ultimately, successful gene therapy may rely on combination therapy. Indeed, a recently designed shRNA targeting Bcl-xl, TERT and VEGF safely suppressed tumor growth by over 90% in a mouse HNSCC model [53].

Corrective Gene Therapy

Oncogenes regulate cell growth and differentiation. Mutations in oncogenes activate them to drive cell growth and realize their oncogenic potential. More than 1% of all the genes in the human genome are oncogenes [2]. Tumor suppressor genes are also ubiquitous with mutations resulting in unregulated cell growth. In cancers, 90% of oncogenes or tumor suppressor genes demonstrate somatic mutations, 20% show germline mutations and 10% show both [55]. Blocking the effect of oncogenes or, contrastingly, enhancing the effect of tumor suppressor genes could potentially revolutionize cancer treatment.

The tumor suppressor gene p53 is mutated in 40–60% of HNSCC and is associated with a poor prognosis, recurrence and resistance to chemoradiation [56–58]. The presence of genomic damage results in p53-mediated cell cycle arrest and, in the case of persisting damage, induction of apoptosis to prevent the propagation of genetic aberrations [3]. Adenovirus vectors have been used to restore p53 function and are able to safely induce HNSCC apoptosis and regression in vitro and in vivo, and are also able to sensitize cancers to chemotherapy or radiation [58–61]. These findings led to the design of p53-containing recombinant adenovirus vectors (Ad-p53) which have since been developed into products – Advexin and Gendicine – that are safe for human use with no dose-limiting toxicity. Fever and/or injection site pain are the primary adverse effects [58]. Gendicine has been approved in China for the treatment of advanced head and neck cancers in conjunction with radiation [58]. In a study of advanced laryngeal cancer treated with Ad-p53 intratumoral monotherapy, 11 of 12 patients showed no evidence of relapse 5 years post-treatment [62]. A phase II study of 69 patients with advanced stage III or IV head and neck cancers demonstrated a 96% overall response rate (64% complete and 32% partial responses) in the Gendicine with radiotherapy arm versus 80% overall response rate (19% complete and 61% partial responses) in the radiotherapy alone arm [63]. Ongoing trials utilizing Advexin and incorporating a comparative chemotherapy arm will be reported in the near future and will further clarify the clinical utility of p53-directed gene therapy.

Immune Modulation Gene Therapy

Enhancing the immune response directed against cancer cells is particularly attractive because: (1) the inherent specificity of the immune system should reduce toxicity against normal cells, (2) the immune response may eradicate metastatic disease, and (3) the generation of immune memory should prevent disease recurrence [3].

One approach involves the stimulation of tumor-infiltrating lymphocytes (TIL), CD8 cytotoxic T cells that are able to recognize tumor-associated antigens and kill cells that harbor them. Early studies demonstrated that the IL-2 gene could be transferred directly into a patient's tumor inducing the formation of local TIL. An excisional biopsy of a draining lymph node was then performed and sensitized TIL extracted. These were propagated in culture and infused back into the patient resulting in eradication of locoregional and distant disease [64]. A second approach involves the transfer of genes encoding major histocompatibility complex (MHC) class I into tumor cells. Many cancers lack class I MHC preventing their recognition by cytotoxic T cells and the resulting generation of an antitumor immune response [3]. In one clinical trial, the use of a cationic liposome to deliver the gene encoding class I MHC HLA-B7 into HNSCC stabilized disease or induced partial responses [65].

Transfer of cytokines such as interferon-γ, GM-CSF and interleukins into tumors using a range of viral vectors has been shown to enhance the host immune response against melanoma but no clinical trials demonstrating significant efficacy or improved survival have been reported [3]. The antitumor cytokine, tumor necrosis factor-α (TNFα) has a potent, tumor-selective apoptotic effect mediated by cellular receptors. However, systemic administration of TNFα induces dose-limiting hypotension and efforts have been directed at inducing a safer, local effect. TNFerade is an adenovirus vector with the TNFα gene inserted downstream of a radiation-induced growth promoter. Gene expression is controlled through radiation and, critically, is localized to the tumor. Intratumoral administration of TNFerade followed by radiation has been shown to induce complete responses in a range of solid tumors including melanoma [66].

Conclusions

An increased understanding of the molecular basis of head and neck cancer has resulted in the development of novel gene therapy approaches. Clinical trials have only recently begun to demonstrate the potential for gene therapy as a low-toxicity, high-efficacy option for the treatment of cancer. The development of these gene therapy options will likely grow in parallel with an increasing knowledge of the precise molecular defects that characterize particular cancers. Numerous challenges still exist in the areas of vector delivery and refinement of the mechanisms regulating gene expression. In the short term, the greatest benefit from gene therapy will likely be derived through combination treatment with existing standard therapies such as radiation or chemotherapy. Ultimately, a range of gene therapy treatments may become available that obviate the need for standard treatments, with the choice of therapy based upon the molecular make up of an individual patient's specific cancer. This 'personalized' gene therapy has the potential to revolutionize the treatment of head and neck cancer in the coming decade and will, hopefully, confer a significant survival benefit.

References

1 Aiuti A, et al: Correction of ADA-SCID by stem cell gene therapy combined with nonmyeloablative conditioning. Science 2002;296:2410–2413.

2 Chisholm E, et al: Gene therapy in head and neck cancer: a review. Postgrad Med J 2007;83:731–737.

3 Harrington KJ, Nutting CM, Pandha HS: Gene therapy for head and neck cancer. Cancer Metastasis Rev 2005;24:147–164.

4 National Cancer Institute Surveillance Epidemiology and End Results. 1973–2006.

5 Capecchi MR: High efficiency transformation by direct microinjection of DNA into cultured mammalian cells. Cell 1980;22:479–488.

6 Heinzerling L, et al: Intratumoral injection of DNA encoding human interleukin 12 into patients with metastatic melanoma: clinical efficacy. Hum Gene Ther 2005;16:35–48.

7 Walther W, et al: Novel jet-injection technology for nonviral intratumoral gene transfer in patients with melanoma and breast cancer. Clin Cancer Res 2008; 14:7545–7553.

8 Yang NS, et al: In vivo and in vitro gene transfer to mammalian somatic cells by particle bombardment. Proc Natl Acad Sci USA 1990;87:9568–9572.

9 Daud AI, et al: Phase I trial of interleukin-12 plasmid electroporation in patients with metastatic melanoma. J Clin Oncol 2008;26:5896–5903.

10 O'Malley BW Jr, et al: Combination nonviral interleukin-2 gene immunotherapy for head and neck cancer: from bench top to bedside. Laryngoscope 2005;115:391–404.

11 Yoo GH, et al: Phase I trial of intratumoral liposome E1A gene therapy in patients with recurrent breast and head and neck cancer. Clin Cancer Res 2001;7:1237–1245.

12 Villaret D, et al: A multicenter phase II study of tgDCC-E1A for the intratumoral treatment of patients with recurrent head and neck squamous cell carcinoma. Head Neck 2002;24:661–669.

13 Sikes ML, et al: In vivo gene transfer into rabbit thyroid follicular cells by direct DNA injection. Hum Gene Ther 1994; 5:837–844.
14 Wolff JA, et al: Direct gene transfer into mouse muscle in vivo. Science 1990;247:1465–1468.
15 Li D, et al: Novel adenoviral gene delivery system targeted against head and neck cancer. Laryngoscope 2008;118: 650–658.
16 Keith WN, et al: Drug insight: Cancer cell immortality-telomerase as a target for novel cancer gene therapies. Nat Clin Pract Oncol 2004;1:88–96.
17 Patel MM, et al: Clinical usefulness of telomerase activation and telomere length in head and neck cancer. Head Neck 2002;24:1060–1067.
18 Hacein-Bey-Abina S, et al: LMO2-associated clonal T cell proliferation in two patients after gene therapy for SCID-X1. Science 2003;302:415–419.
19 Kohn DB: Gene therapy for childhood immunological diseases. Bone Marrow Transplant 2008;41:199–205.
20 Barzon L, et al: Gene therapy of thyroid cancer via retrovirally-driven combined expression of human interleukin-2 and herpes simplex virus thymidine kinase. Eur J Endocrinol 2003;148:73–80.
21 Chawla SP, et al: Advanced phase I/II studies of targeted gene delivery in vivo: intravenous Rexin-G for gemcitabine-resistant metastatic pancreatic cancer. Mol Ther 2010;18:435–441.
22 Aiuti A, et al: Gene therapy for immunodeficiency due to adenosine deaminase deficiency. N Engl J Med 2009;360:447–458.
23 Ott MG, et al: Correction of X-linked chronic granulomatous disease by gene therapy, augmented by insertional activation of MDS1-EVI1, PRDM16 or SETBP1. Nat Med 2006;12:401–409.
24 Brody SL, Crystal RG: Adenovirus-mediated in vivo gene transfer. Ann NY Acad Sci 1994;716:90–101; discussion 101–103.
25 O'Malley BW Jr, et al: Adenovirus-mediated gene therapy for human head and neck squamous cell cancer in a nude mouse model. Cancer Res 1995;55: 1080–1085.
26 Flotte TR: Gene therapy: the first two decades and the current state-of-the-art. J Cell Physiol 2007;213:301–305.
27 Raper SE, et al: Fatal systemic inflammatory response syndrome in a ornithine transcarbamylase deficient patient following adenoviral gene transfer. Mol Genet Metab 2003;80:148–158.
28 Engelhardt JF, et al: Ablation of E2A in recombinant adenoviruses improves transgene persistence and decreases inflammatory response in mouse liver. Proc Natl Acad Sci USA 1994;91: 6196–6200.
29 Samulski RJ, Chang LS, Shenk T: Helper-free stocks of recombinant adeno-associated viruses: normal integration does not require viral gene expression. J Virol 1989;63:3822–3828.
30 Varghese S, Rabkin SD: Oncolytic herpes simplex virus vectors for cancer virotherapy. Cancer Gene Ther 2002;9: 967–978.
31 Chahlavi A, et al: Replication-competent herpes simplex virus vector G207 and cisplatin combination therapy for head and neck squamous cell carcinoma. Neoplasia 1999;1:162–169.
32 Hu JC, et al: A phase I study of OncoVEXGM-CSF, a second-generation oncolytic herpes simplex virus expressing granulocyte macrophage colony-stimulating factor. Clin Cancer Res 2006; 12:6737–6747.
33 Fire A, et al: Potent and specific genetic interference by double-stranded RNA in Caenorhabditis elegans. Nature 1998;391:806–811.
34 Behlke MA: Progress towards in vivo use of siRNAs. Mol Ther 2006;13:644–670.
35 Kim DH, Rossi JJ: Strategies for silencing human disease using RNA interference. Nat Rev Genet 2007;8:173–184.
36 Morrissey DV, et al: Potent and persistent in vivo anti-HBV activity of chemically modified siRNAs. Nat Biotechnol 2005;23:1002–1007.
37 Higuchi Y, Kawakami S, Hashida M: Strategies for in vivo delivery of siRNAs: recent progress. BioDrugs 2010;24: 195–205.
38 Schiffelers RM, et al: Cancer siRNA therapy by tumor selective delivery with ligand-targeted sterically stabilized nanoparticle. Nucleic Acids Res 2004;32: e149.
39 Hagstrom JE, et al: A facile nonviral method for delivering genes and siRNAs to skeletal muscle of mammalian limbs. Mol Ther 2004;10:386–398.
40 Karagiannis TC, El-Osta A: RNA interference and potential therapeutic applications of short interfering RNAs. Cancer Gene Ther 2005;12:787–795.
41 Xu F, et al: Phase I and biodistribution study of recombinant adenovirus vector-mediated herpes simplex virus thymidine kinase gene and ganciclovir administration in patients with head and neck cancer and other malignant tumors. Cancer Gene Ther 2009;16:723–730.
42 Saito K, et al: Cytotoxicity and antiangiogenesis by fibroblast growth factor 2-targeted Ad-TK cancer gene therapy. Laryngoscope 2009;119:665–674.
43 Nemunaitis J, et al: Pilot trial of intravenous infusion of a replication-selective adenovirus (ONYX-015) in combination with chemotherapy or IL-2 treatment in refractory cancer patients. Cancer Gene Ther 2003;10:341–352.
44 Nemunaitis J, et al: Selective replication and oncolysis in p53 mutant tumors with ONYX-015, an E1B-55kD gene-deleted adenovirus, in patients with advanced head and neck cancer: a phase II trial. Cancer Res 2000;60:6359–6366.
45 Nemunaitis J, et al: Phase II trial of intratumoral administration of ONYX-015, a replication-selective adenovirus, in patients with refractory head and neck cancer. J Clin Oncol 2001;19:289–298.
46 Khuri FR, et al: a controlled trial of intratumoral ONYX-015, a selectively-replicating adenovirus, in combination with cisplatin and 5-fluorouracil in patients with recurrent head and neck cancer. Nat Med 2000;6:879–885.
47 Xia ZJ, et al: Phase III randomized clinical trial of intratumoral injection of E1B gene-deleted adenovirus (H101) combined with cisplatin-based chemotherapy in treating squamous cell cancer of head and neck or esophagus. Ai Zheng 2004;23:1666–1670.
48 Kurihara Y, et al: Telomerase-specific virotheranostics for human head and neck cancer. Clin Cancer Res 2009;15: 2335–2343.
49 Abuzeid WM, et al: Molecular disruption of RAD50 sensitizes human tumor cells to cisplatin-based chemotherapy. J Clin Invest 2009;119:1974–1985.
50 Hanahan D, Folkman J: Patterns and emerging mechanisms of the angiogenic switch during tumorigenesis. Cell 1996; 86:353–364.
51 Hanahan D, Weinberg RA: The hallmarks of cancer. Cell 2000;100:57–70.

52 Teknos TN, et al: Elevated serum vascular endothelial growth factor and decreased survival in advanced laryngeal carcinoma. Head Neck 2002;24:1004–1011.
53 Chen SM, et al: Effect of blocking VEGF, hTERT and Bcl-xl by multiple shRNA expression vectors on the human laryngeal squamous carcinoma xenograft in nude mice. Cancer Biol Ther 2008;7:734–739.
54 Wang Y, et al: Application of combination of short hairpin RNA segments for silencing VEGF, TERT and Bcl-xl expression in laryngeal squamous carcinoma. Cancer Biol Ther 2008;7:896–901.
55 Futreal PA, et al: A census of human cancer genes. Nat Rev Cancer 2004;4:177–183.
56 Koch WM, et al: p53 mutation and locoregional treatment failure in head and neck squamous cell carcinoma. J Natl Cancer Inst 1996;88:1580–1586.
57 Brachman DG, et al: Occurrence of p53 gene deletions and human papilloma virus infection in human head and neck cancer. Cancer Res 1992;52:4832–4836.
58 Huang PI, et al: Targeted genetic and viral therapy for advanced head and neck cancers. Drug Discov Today 2009;14:570–578.
59 Clayman GL, et al: In vivo molecular therapy with p53 adenovirus for microscopic residual head and neck squamous carcinoma. Cancer Res 1995;55:1–6.
60 Liu TJ, et al: Growth suppression of human head and neck cancer cells by the introduction of a wild-type p53 gene via a recombinant adenovirus. Cancer Res 1994;54:3662–3667.
61 Zhang WW, et al: Safety evaluation of Ad5CMV-p53 in vitro and in vivo. Hum Gene Ther 1995;6:155–164.
62 Han DM, et al: Effectiveness of recombinant adenovirus p53 injection on laryngeal cancer: phase I clinical trial and follow up. Zhonghua Yi Xue Za Zhi 2003;83:2029–2032.
63 Zhang SW, et al: Recombinant adenovirus-p53 gene therapy combined with radiotherapy for head and neck squamous-cell carcinoma. Zhonghua Zhong Liu Za Zhi 2005;27:426–428.
64 Immunization of cancer patients using autologous cancer cells modified by insertion of the gene for interleukin-2. Hum Gene Ther 1992;3:75–90.
65 Gleich LL, et al: Clinical experience with HLA-B7 plasmid DNA/lipid complex in advanced squamous cell carcinoma of the head and neck. Arch Otolaryngol Head Neck Surg 2001;127:775–779.
66 McLoughlin JM, et al: TNFerade, an adenovector carrying the transgene for human tumor necrosis factor alpha, for patients with advanced solid tumors: surgical experience and long-term follow-up. Ann Surg Oncol 2005;12:825–830.

Waleed M. Abuzeid, MD
University of Michigan Health System, Department of Otolaryngology
1904 Taubman Center, 1500 E. Medical Center Dr.
Ann Arbor, MI 48109 (USA)
Tel. +1 267 266 5302, Fax +1 734 936 8052

Author Index

Subject Index